The Ethics of Caring for Ol[der]

Second Edition

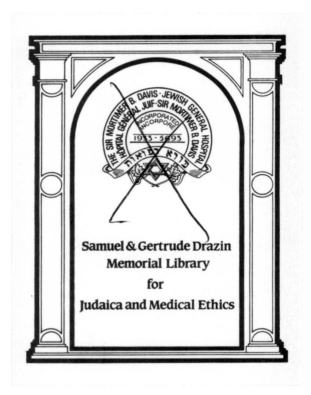
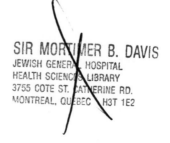

The Ethics of Caring for Older People

Written and researched by: Ann Sommerville and Danielle Hamm
With contributions from: Caroline Harrison, Julian Sheather
Editorial assistant: Tricia Fraser

We would like to thank all the individuals and organisations who
generously gave advice, especially:

Chris Chaloner, Pauline Ford and Ann Gallagher, Royal College of Nursing;
Helen Clarke, the English Law Society;
Jan Dewing, Honorary Research Fellow, University of Ulster;
Juliet Dunmore and members of the BMA's Patient Liaison Group;
Mark Henaghan, Dean of Law Faculty, University of Otago, New Zealand;
Michael Keegan, General Medical Council;
Brian Livingstone, Scottish Government;
Susan Lockhart and Hugh Donald, Shepherd and Wedderburn LLP;
Donald Lyons, Director, Mental Welfare Commission for Scotland;
Francis Lyons, Capsticks;
Helena McKeown and members of the BMA's Community Care Committee;
Theresa Mann, Senior Palliative Care Nurse, Imperial College NHS Trust;
Medical Ethics Committee of the BMA;
Jacqueline Morris, David Oliver, Alex Mair and Ian Donald, British Geriatric Association;
Tom Owen, City University and Help the Aged;
Fiona Randall, Consultant in Palliative Medicine, Royal Bournemouth and Christchurch
Hospitals;
Lucy Sutton and Simon Chapman, National Council for Palliative Care;
Beverley Taylor, Official Solicitor's Office;
Ginny Wright, Consultant in Elderly Medicine, Charing Cross Hospital.

The Ethics of Caring for Older People

SECOND EDITION

British Medical Association

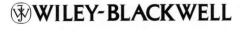

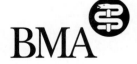

A John Wiley & Sons, Ltd., Publication

This edition first published 2009, © 2009 British Medical Association

BMJ Books is an imprint of BMJ Publishing Group Limited, used under licence by Blackwell Publishing which was acquired by John Wiley & Sons in February 2007. Blackwell's publishing programme has been merged with Wiley's global Scientific, Technical and Medical business to form Wiley-Blackwell.

Registered office: John Wiley & Sons Ltd, The Atrium, Southern Gate, Chichester, West Sussex, PO19 8SQ, UK

Editorial offices: 9600 Garsington Road, Oxford, OX4 2DQ, UK
The Atrium, Southern Gate, Chichester, West Sussex, PO19 8SQ, UK
111 River Street, Hoboken, NJ 07030-5774, USA

For details of our global editorial offices, for customer services and for information about how to apply for permission to reuse the copyright material in this book please see our website at www.wiley.com/wiley-blackwell

Library of Congress Cataloging-in-Publication Data
The ethics of caring for older people / British Medical Association. — 2nd ed.
    p. ; cm
    Rev. ed. of: The older person : consent and care : report of the British Medical Association and the Royal College of Nursing. 1995.
    Includes bibliographical references and index.
    ISBN: 978-1-4051-7627-9
    1. Older people—Medical care—Moral and ethical aspects—Great Britain.
2. Informed consent (Medical law)—Great Britain. 3. Advance directives (Medical care)—Great Britain.
4. Patient refusal of treatment—Great Britian. 5. Refusal to treat—Great Britain. I. British Medical Association. II. Older person.
    [DNLM: 1. Health Services for the Aged—ethics. 2. Aged. 3. Informed Consent—ethics.
4. Nursing Care—ethics. 5. Patient Rights—ethics. WT 31 E856 2009]
    RA564.8.E934 2009
    174.2'9073—dc22

ISBN: 978-1-4051-7627-9

A catalogue record for this book is available from the British Library.

Set in 9.5/12 Minion Regular by Charon Tec Ltd (A Macmillan Company), Chennai, India
Printed and bound in Malaysia by KHL Printing Co Sdn Bhd

Contents

Executive summary

This report is mainly about communicating well with older people who are receiving health care and respecting their decisions. It challenges stereotypes and encourages a consistently individualised approach. Chapter 1 spells out the remit, which is to focus on the law and ethics of consent, refusal and confidentiality in the care of older people. Chapters 2 and 3 look at how key information is communicated so that older people can make properly informed choices. Among the things that older people often complain about are the lack of attention given to their views and the inadequate information provided to them about their health care options.

Most older people are willing and competent to decide for themselves but some experience mental impairment. Across most of the United Kingdom, there have been significant legal changes in the way in which health care decisions are made on behalf of adults who cannot decide for themselves. (The terms 'capacity' and 'competence' mean the same thing and are used interchangeably here.) All adults are assumed to have this ability unless there is evidence to the contrary. This is discussed in Chapter 4, which sets out the law regarding care and treatment decisions for people whose mental ability is impaired and describes the legal changes, relating to proxy consent and the role of advocates. The law and ethics specifically relating to medical treatment decisions by individuals themselves in advance of their loss of mental capacity is dealt with in Chapter 7.

By mutual agreement, relatives often play a large role in the health care decisions made by older people but it cannot be assumed that this is always what the older person wants. Chapter 5 deals in detail with confidentiality and management of health information, including when and how it can be disclosed to relatives and others. Another area in which assumptions cannot be made concerns the use of so-called protective measures for older people, such as bed rails and locked doors to prevent confused people from wandering. Measures originally intended to prevent harm can be perpetuated as a way of compensating for staff shortages by effectively depriving older people of their freedom of movement. Such deprivation of liberty can be an offence under human rights legislation. Chapter 6 looks at the importance of consent and refusal in this context and also broaches the issue of the covert medication of older people.

Communication and choices at the end of life are discussed in Chapter 8 which flags up how advance planning and truthful information can help people retain some control. It also emphasises the importance of not giving dying people and their relatives unrealistic expectations about what can be achieved in terms of controlling the dying process. Difficult decisions about treatment withdrawal and attempting resuscitation after cardiac arrest are also discussed in this chapter.

Themes such as honesty, empathy and treating older people as individuals run throughout the book. Older people have the same rights as anyone else but are frequently treated differently. On the one hand, they often experience exclusion and marginalisation from mainstream society and, on the other, overprotective attitudes which discourage them from taking risks or discussing their feelings about sensitive topics such as death and bereavement. Most of the advice in the report applies equally to all patient groups but endemic ageist attitudes in society can create a blind spot in the provision of care to older people. Avoiding ageism, including through communication training, is emphasised for care providers.

There is some overlap between chapters in the expectation that readers may dip into sections for specific advice rather than necessarily read the book in its entirety.

Chapter 1 **Introduction**

Scope and purpose of this report

Unless we are already old, we will be the old people of the future and so we all have an interest in ensuring that older people's rights are properly respected. The remit of this report is narrow. It concentrates specifically on the rights of older people to have information and be consulted in decisions about their care and medical treatment, including how their confidentiality is protected. If they become mentally incompetent, their former wishes must feature as part of any judgement about their 'best interests'. These may appear very simple and mundane issues but they affect every single transaction between care providers and older people and contribute to the general culture within which care and treatment are provided to this population. The report is mainly aimed at health professionals but many of the problems will also be familiar to people providing other kinds of care and support, and so the advice may be useful to them too.

The rights to accept or refuse treatment and have one's confidentiality protected are important to everyone but older people are more likely than others to have those rights ignored. Nevertheless, there is a risk that focussing only on the older generation could reinforce the notion that they are somehow different. The reality is that they are already treated differently, despite the fact that adults' rights are not age-related. For health professionals, the same obligations apply regardless of who the patient is but specific guidance is needed for this group of people because:
- the risks of receiving inadequate care increase with age;
- offers of treatment options also diminish; older people are less likely to be offered specialist care than younger people, especially at the end of life;
- inadequate discussion and explanation of treatment options are more likely;
- older people are often seen as stereotypes rather than as individuals;
- they are marginalised in discussion if their hearing or memory problems lead professionals to deal primarily with their carers or relatives;
- they often lack confidence to insist on their rights or question what is proposed.

The Ethics of Caring for Older People 2nd Edition. By British Medical Association.
Published 2009 by Blackwell Publishing Limited, ISBN: 9781405176279.

Older people are treated differently in ways which disadvantage them. In 2007, for example, the Parliamentary Joint Committee on Human Rights flagged up a range of areas where older individuals endure discrimination and neglect in health services. It called for 'an entire culture change' (Ref. [1], p. 3). This report seeks to tease out how a culture change might begin by illustrating best practice in relation to frank and effective communication, consent and patient confidentiality. It also highlights some assumptions about older people that need to be challenged.

The difference in approach to older people is often subtle and nuanced rather than dramatic. In many cases, the differing attitudes pass without comment since they reflect broadly held perceptions and prejudices within society. Terminology can be crucial. By labelling people as 'vulnerable', for example, society not only encourages a different and more protective attitude towards them but can also give the erroneous impression that they are less able mentally to decide for themselves. Legally and ethically, everyone should be assumed to have the ability to decide for themselves unless there is evidence to the contrary. This includes people with a diagnosed mental impairment who can often make some decisions themselves, even if they need support deciding complex matters. In reality, all people are vulnerable in one way or another. Illness, disability, bereavement or other mental distress render individuals more so, and, as people age, they are more at risk of these effects. Yet many older people live healthy, independent lives without much contact with health services. The focus here, however, is mainly on those who need treatment, care or support due to ill health, a learning disability, mental illness or loss of mental capacity. Some may be unable to make valid decisions for themselves.

Older people are often perceived as stereotypes and those from minority groups, such as those who are gay, lesbian or from an ethnic minority, have the double burden of stereotyping. Health and care professionals know that communicating and building relationships on an individual basis are important for quality care but these activities are also time-consuming. It is essential that negative stereotypes are avoided as they are immensely undermining, especially when accompanied by the presumption that age itself is a sickness. If it is assumed that frailty and degeneration are inevitable aspects of age, individuals presenting with treatable conditions will not be offered treatment. Symptoms are dismissed as normal for older people in situations where younger people would routinely be referred for investigation. Older people are less frequently referred to specialist services. Appropriate treatment options, including their risks and drawbacks, are often not discussed with them.

All patients facing serious illness or entering hospital encounter a power imbalance between themselves and the professionals caring for them. They may be reluctant to question staff or feel hesitant about asserting their rights. The regulatory body for doctors, the General Medical Council, emphasises that a good doctor–patient relationship is 'a partnership based on openness, trust and good communication'[2] but older people say they often feel bypassed in their interchanges with health professionals. Sometimes, this perception of being 'written off' or 'fobbed off' is because they are not given frank answers about their prognosis and options, especially when the information is distressing. In institutional settings, older people appear more at risk of being given sedatives or other drugs without any proper discussion of why they need them or whether they would prefer to do without. This report is partly about the attitudes with which care providers approach older people who are sometimes treated as though they have impaired mental abilities even when they are mentally competent. Some older people, however, do suffer from cognitive impairment and, in Chapter 4, this report sets out the legal changes which apply to such patients. In England, Wales and Scotland, the mental capacity legislation affects decision-making for patients who cannot decide for themselves and many older people will be affected by it. In Northern Ireland, such issues remain a matter of common law. This is also covered in Chapter 4.

Who is the report for?

The report seeks to reinforce best practice among primary care providers, outreach teams, care home staff, geriatric care teams and patient advocates. Non-health professionals providing support to older clients living independently, with relatives, in care homes, hospitals or hospices may also find it helpful.

Who is the report about?

Attempting to make generalisations about a large slice of the population on the basis of age alone is likely to be unhelpful. According to some public documents, the older population encompasses everyone over the age of 65 but the differences between people in their 60s and those in their 90s can be just as pronounced as between a thirty-something and a sixty year old. Old age is a relative concept and the fact that people are living longer and fitter lives affects whom we perceive as the 'older person'. In 1901, when the average life expectancy was in the 40s, 50 seemed relatively old but as average life expectancy has virtually doubled, 50 seems relatively young. Old age has no start date. 'Some people decide to be old at 65, when they "retire", which rightly sounds like walking backwards, out of sight. Some of us suddenly realise, perhaps at 80, that we have become old (Ref. [3], p. 3).' Whilst it is important to remember that older people are not an homogenous group, as a population they are more likely to be living with disability, depression and multiple health problems. They often experience social isolation, poor support networks, poverty and discrimination on the basis of their age. Although they have more contact with care providers, the roots of many of their problems are social. Underlying social isolation often remains unaddressed.

Rather than asking when does somebody become 'old', it is more useful to ask what is particularly relevant about being old? In the context of this report, we use the term 'older person' or 'older patient' as shorthand for people at the stage of life where they increasingly need assistance to look after themselves. We are not talking about everyone within a predetermined age group but rather considering how individuals – at varying chronological ages – start to experience frailty and a need for support. This experience is one of subtle but multiple losses and transitions. Friends, contemporaries and loved ones die. Health problems and sensory impairments increase older people's sense of social exclusion, as do mobility problems and the loss of independence if they have to give up driving. Although there are some obvious correlations between increasing age and need for assistance, the experience of vulnerability rather than age markers alone are what defines the 'older person' in this report. Clearly, all patients should be treated as individuals but older patients are more likely to be stereotyped rather than treated as individuals. This can lead to unfair discrimination.

Specific ethical principles most relevant to older patients

Sound ethical principles, such as respect for patient autonomy and confidentiality, acting in a patient's best interests, avoiding harm and showing empathy, apply to all patients equally. In addition, ethical guidance concerning the care of older people needs to focus on:

- *being person-centred and holistic since older individuals often have multiple problems and needs;*
- *being mindful of patients' dignity and safeguarding their privacy;*
- *promoting individuals' independence, quality of life and ability to exercise control;*
- *being sensitive to issues of justice and not discriminating unfairly on grounds of age;*
- *respecting different cultural values;*
- *recognising societal factors that affect our behaviour and attitudes towards older people.*

These values are important for all patients but inherent ageism within society often causes us to listen and respond to the views of older people differently in comparison with how we react to younger people. We are less likely to listen, more likely to make assumptions, and more likely to overlook treatable health problems or to normalise them as just being part of ageing. Supporting older people to make informed decisions is often more time-consuming and challenging than offering options to other groups and so is more often overlooked.

Person-centred holistic care

Older people have a wide range of care needs and often have multiple morbidity. They often need multidisciplinary care. This needs to be well co-ordinated so looking at problems in isolation should be avoided. Factual information about an individual's diagnosis, prognosis and underlying pathology needs to be discussed with that person, including the risks associated with treatment options. Good communication between different care providers is also essential but needs to be balanced with respect for patient confidentiality. In hospital, older people are usually treated in general wards where staff may have had only a minimum of training in caring for such patients. As inpatients and in the community, older people's health care is often focussed on the most obvious physical problems, so that conditions such as depression are under-diagnosed. Factual information about a patient's psychological state is often not sought and problems which seriously impinge on quality of life, such as anxiety, insomnia or failing cognitive abilities, frequently go unexplored. Sometimes this is due to the care provider's view that these are a natural part of the human condition in older life.

Respect for dignity and privacy

Older people are often the focus of attention for a range of health and social care professionals for fleeting snatches of time in which various activities have to be compressed. They may be asked to discuss personal aspects of their life or health in front of other people, such as whether they can go to the lavatory by themselves or suffer from constipation. Sometimes questions are addressed to the relatives as if the older person were incompetent. Among the common frustrations expressed by older patients are:
• being addressed in an inappropriate manner;
• being spoken about as if they were not there;
• not being given proper information;
• not seeking their consent or not considering their wishes;
• being placed in mixed sex accommodation without adequate privacy[4].

Promoting independence and quality of life

Health care and social support aim to maximise individuals' ability to function and enjoy life. For many people, feelings of self-worth are linked to social or professional networks or the family. If no longer engaged in social activities or as a result of bereavement and losses within their peer group, older people risk becoming socially and emotionally isolated. They may see themselves in a negative light if lacking social interaction with other people and suffer low self-esteem. This is often reinforced by negative attitudes within society. Feeling undervalued or inept at coping can lead older people to become more dependent and stop trying to do things for themselves. Good quality health care and social support – when needed – aim to promote independence and help people maintain their quality of life. Exercising choice where they can assumes more importance for older people as control over other aspects of life becomes more elusive. The writer, Richard Hoggart, described life in his 80s, saying how 'relatively small matters annoy more because they seem to be indicators of a growing loss of everyday intuitive control, physical and mental' (Ref. [3], p. 12).

Empowering people to keep control, however, can also give rise to dilemmas, such as the degree to which any person has the freedom to take risks. Even though older people are entitled to the same freedom as others to risk their health by unwise choices, society often displays a particularly protective or paternalistic attitude to them. Care providers feel more professionally responsible and subject to greater moral obligations when caring for patients who are physically vulnerable. Failing to prevent foreseeable harm occurring to them is seen as more culpable, even if the individual desires to remain independent and take risks. Among the typical scenarios raised by health professionals are cases where older people choose to live independently alone or in an isolated setting, rather than in sheltered housing, after they have had falls and fractures. Respecting their choice to continue with a risky course of action may shorten their life and incur additional health care costs. Nevertheless, it is important that the informed choices of older people are as respected as those of any other group in society. Rather than overruling an older person for his or her 'own good', it is important that families and care providers discuss with the individual how risks can be minimised and reasonable steps taken to prevent accidents.

Justice and non-discrimination

Care providers have duties to avoid discriminating unfairly against some patients or groups of patients. They also have a professional and ethical duty to ensure that treatment decisions are made on the basis of a proper assessment of the relevant factors in each individual case. Decisions cannot be based on assumptions about the patient's age or disability. Everyone is entitled to a fair and unprejudiced assessment of his or her individual situation and the Human Rights Act (1998) provides all patients being cared for by a public authority, including all NHS and local authority-run facilities, with redress against unfair discrimination in health matters. In 2008, the government pledged to extend the Act to afford protection to publicly funded residents in privately run residential and nursing homes. Prior to that, in 2007, the Parliamentary Human Rights Committee highlighted the need to address discrimination against older people in hospitals and care homes where they were said to suffer neglect and lack of respect for their privacy[1]. Also in 2007, the Commission for Equality, Diversity and Human Rights assumed responsibility for enforcing equality law in England, Scotland and Wales. Part of its role is to identify unfair discrimination and encourage best practice in the way vulnerable people are treated.

Respecting differing cultural values

Ensuring that people are treated as individuals requires that some attention be given to their own values, expectations and cultural background. In a multicultural society, such as the United Kingdom, people have a diversity of attitudes on matters such as personal autonomy. In families where the head or the eldest son commonly expects to make decisions on behalf of other family members, and they expect that too, tensions can arise when health professionals encourage individuals to make choices independently. Care providers must ensure that the patient's rights are not overridden by well-intentioned relatives but sensitivity is also needed to ascertain the individual's genuine preference. In some cases, older people voluntarily choose to defer to the views of a close relative. Some work has been done in New Zealand about formally considering different cultural expectations regarding individual consent. A code of rights states everyone's rights to services that take into account their needs, values and beliefs. It recognises that these might differ between cultural, religious, social and ethnic groups. In this context, respecting cultural rights applies primarily to the manner in which people are approached to give their views rather than diluting the requirement for them to give informed consent if they are competent. For example, if it is culturally appropriate for a wide group to be present when a decision is made or to be informed of what is happening and the individual agrees with that way of doing things, discussion should be arranged in that way. The decision would still ultimately be for the individual patient. The group cannot make the decision for the patient but should be consulted and able to offer advice, if that is the patient's choice. Thus the cultural issues may well affect the manner of communication without altering the basic premise of individual patient choice.

Like other patients, older people should be encouraged to understand the implications of their medical condition and the choices open to them. They may want family support in coming to a decision but the choice of who to involve in decision-making, and to what degree, should rest with the patient. Relatives cannot be allowed to remove the choice by, for example, attempting to prohibit care providers from engaging in discussion with the patient, even though the family often influences the ultimate decision.

Recognising societal factors affect our behaviour and attitudes

Ageism is common in society and constitutes a bias on the basis of age alone, regardless of other factors such as a person's skills, ability and experience. It is as unacceptable as any other prejudice but can be more subtle than overt. Attention has been drawn to how 'too many NHS staff are prone to ageism and reluctant to work with the elderly'[5], a prejudice that would be promptly condemned if applied to patients with disabilities or different racial backgrounds. The government has tried to address the problem by measures such as the National Service Framework for Older People (2001), which required that ageism be eliminated from health and care services. The 2006 review of the Framework[6] concluded that whilst there was a general reduction in explicit discrimination and age-related policies, older people were still treated with a lack of dignity and respect in hospitals. The report called upon central government to develop a cross-developmental programme to shape more positive attitudes towards ageing.

Summary of chapter

- *The fundamental message is to treat older people as individuals like any other group and attempt to avoid assumptions about their wants, needs or abilities.*
- *Unconscious ageism can be difficult to tackle because it emerges in various guises. It may not be embodied in explicit policies but in negative attitudes towards older people which are harder to eliminate.*
- *Well-intentioned but overly-protective paternalism is a form of ageism as is the failure to offer older people information about their health, medication and treatment options.*
- *Age discrimination is also perpetrated through policies which may not explicitly exclude people on the basis of age but disproportionately affect older people.*

References

1. House of Lords, House of Commons, Joint Committee on Human Rights (2007). *The Human Rights of Older People in Healthcare, Eighteenth Report of Session 2006–07. Volume 1 – Report and Formal Minutes.* The Stationery Office Ltd, London.
2. General Medical Council (2008). *Consent: Patients and Doctors Making Decisions Together.* GMC, London.
3. Hoggart R (2005). *Promises to Keep: Thoughts in Old Age.* Continuum, London.
4. Healthcare Commission (2007). *Caring for Dignity: A National Report on Dignity in Care for Older People while in Hospital.* Commission for Healthcare Audit and Inspection, London.
5. Oliver D (2007). Geriatric medicine: changing staff attitudes. *Health Service Journal* 22/11/2007.
6. Healthcare Commission, the Audit Commission and the Commission for Social Care Inspection (2006). *Living Well in Later Life. A Review of Progress against the National Service Framework for Older People.* Commission for Healthcare Audit and Inspection, London.

Further resources

Department of Health (2001). *National Service Framework for Older People.* DH, London.

Department of Health (2006). *A New Ambition for Old Age: Next Steps in Implementing the National Service Framework for Older People.* DH, London.

Healthcare Commission (2007). *Caring for dignity: A National Report on Dignity in Care for Older People while in Hospital.* Commission for Healthcare Audit and Inspection, London.

House of Lords, House of Commons, Joint Committee on Human Rights (2007). *The Human Rights of Older People in Healthcare, Eighteenth Report of Session 2006–07.* The Stationery Office Ltd, London.

Ros Levenson (2003). *Auditing Age Discrimination. A Practical Approach to Promoting Age Equality in Health and Social Care.* King's Fund, London.

Ros Levenson (2007). *The Challenge of Dignity in Care: Upholding the Rights of the Individual.* Help the Aged, London.

Chapter 2 **Importance of communication and barriers to it**

Most of what needs to be said about good communication applies equally to patients of any age but the assumption often appears to be made that older people have less desire for information or are less able to cope with it. Even when they are mentally competent, it is sometimes assumed that they will be overwhelmed or confused by too much. This may partly be because the current generation of older people grew up in a less questioning period and have lower expectations about their entitlement to information. Age-related losses can also reduce older people's self-esteem, leaving them hesitant about demanding information. In hospitals and residential care homes, staff are often under time constraints which also make it difficult to provide good personalised care, especially to older people who have dementia or other mental health problems and so need more specialised attention.

A 2007 study[1] by the Alzheimer's Society found that many older people with dementia were only given five minutes' attention a day by care home staff who were often insufficiently trained to help them. As a result, such individuals were at risk of being neglected, ignored and excluded from decision-making, even when they could make choices with help. The study also pointed out that people with dementia were over-represented in the group that care staff found most difficult and the least rewarding to care for. Patients living with dementia may be able to decide for themselves if the options are appropriately presented. When they are ignored, however, people with dementia sometimes communicate through challenging behaviour, such as hitting out. Communicating with them is a highly skilled task but, instead of providing trained staff with enough time to talk, the Alzheimer's Society found that managers sometimes rely on sedation to deal with challenging behaviour. Similar criticisms were made by the Commission for Social Care Inspection in 2008[2]. The Commission found some examples of excellent personalised care but also warned that the care system in general, and residential and nursing homes in particular, were often neglecting individuals with dementia.

The presumption must be that all individuals are 'offered' information about their condition and treatment in a manner appropriate to their needs.

The Ethics of Caring for Older People 2nd Edition. By British Medical Association.
Published 2009 by Blackwell Publishing Limited, ISBN: 9781405176279.

This includes people who have a mental impairment but who could participate in decisions, if choices were explained simply. Information should be tailored to their needs by, for example, putting it into pictures. Maintaining social interaction and good communication are facets of ageing well. Health in later life is not only dependent upon physical well-being and ability to function but also upon active involvement with others. Communication with care providers and health professionals is important since there is some evidence that older people both live longer and respond better to health care when they have strong social support networks and communicate closely with professionals[3]. Effective communication is an ethical duty for health professionals but older people often get much less attention. Care providers need to ensure that older patients' hearing or communication difficulties are properly addressed and that relatives do not prevent patients from knowing the facts about their condition. Honesty is a vitally important aspect of treatment decisions for all patients, not least because conflict and disagreement can result from poor communication or inadequate provision of accurate information. For all patients, information should be provided sensitively, especially when the implications are upsetting or when there is medical uncertainty about the future prognosis. Ideally, euphemisms should be avoided, particularly with patients who are likely to be unfamiliar with them, including those whose first language is not English. If euphemisms are used, the implications should be made clear and understandable.

The duty to listen and offer information

A key part of health care is taking patients' history and getting a feel for what they want to know. All patients should be offered information about their condition and treatment options in a sensitive way. Talking to older people and their relatives often involves taboo subjects such as death, delirium, dementia, incontinence and pressure sores, which need to be broached with particular care. They may have unrealistic expectations about what medicine can offer and be shocked by the unpredictable nature of illness, frailty and chronic co-morbidities in older age. Patients become anxious in hospital settings if communication is poor or if it breaks down during long waits or inter-ward transfers. If they are delirious, information from their relatives is crucial to planning their care.

Patients who understand the implications of the treatment options have the right to accept or refuse them (unless it is compulsory treatment under mental health legislation) but failure by health professionals to offer relevant information could invalidate patients' decisions. (The law on this point is discussed in Chapter 4.) Some may not want all the details but need to know basic information, such as:

- the evidence for the diagnosis and prognosis, including the limits of what is known;
- treatment options, including any promising options not available on the NHS;
- the implications, drawbacks and likely side effects of treatment;
- the main alternatives, including non-treatment, and their implications.

In particular, if innovative, risky, painful or very serious procedures are proposed, patients need to be aware of what is involved. The doctors' regulatory body, the General Medical Council (GMC), says that if patients indicate that they want somebody else to decide for them, doctors should explain why it is still important for the patient to understand the options and what is involved[4]. If patients refuse information, doctors are advised by the GMC to find out why. Ultimately if, after discussion, the patient still refuses to have any details, that wish should be respected but the doctor must still give the patient at least the core information so that the person can consent in a valid way to the investigation or treatment.

Case example – effective communication

E was an active person in her late 80s with a good quality of life but with a faulty heart valve which continued to deteriorate, despite medication. She understood that valve replacement was an option and initially regarded it as a solution to all her problems, without fully understanding the risks involved. She felt outraged that health professionals were 'writing her off' when they appeared reluctant to arrange the operation. Her cardiologist needed to explain in clear language the risks and side effects of the procedure, including the risk that E would not survive the surgery and, if she did, it could take up to a year for her to recover her current mobility. During that period, she would be considerably less active and have to adjust to another lifestyle. Without surgery, the heart defect would continue to deteriorate but this would probably be at a relatively slow pace, allowing her to pursue for the foreseeable future the activities she enjoyed. Neither alternative offered an ideal solution. E needed to have enough clear information to weigh up whether it was better for her to continue in her current way of life without surgery or take the risk of a major operation. She also needed reassurance that choosing not to have it would not be seen as a lack of courage on her part or an indication that she was being fobbed off by her doctor. E chose not to have surgery. Through frank discussion with E of the risks involved as well as the benefits, the cardiologist helped her to make the choice with which she felt most comfortable.

If they feel inhibited about questioning health professionals, older people may find it helpful to have written information setting out the facts and the commonly asked queries relating to their condition. Information sheets, including for those whose first language is not English, are not a substitute for discussion but can be helpful. Clear documentation:

- increases patient satisfaction and reduces complaints;
- increases adherence to treatment regimes;
- increases self-care and improves self-management;
- promotes active coping;
- reduces psychological distress and anxiety[5].

Their beliefs, values and cultural backgrounds affect what patients ask and how they handle information. Assumptions should not be made, however, about what they want, based on their age, background or ethnicity. All patients should be encouraged to be involved in decision-making. Deliberate concealment of facts that patients want to know and the covert medication of competent people, constitute an abuse, even if relatives ask for such things. When information is offered, it should be in a way the recipient can best comprehend it, including by signing or through an interpreter. If patients have a diagnosis involving eventual mental impairment, unjustified assumptions are sometimes made about their current abilities so that they are not offered information about their future. Dementia is a case in point. Patient groups, such as the Scottish Dementia Working Group[6], say that the expectations of health professionals appear to be set very low automatically when they talk to people diagnosed with dementia, even before the patient's competence is significantly impaired. The support group, composed of people with dementia, advocates on behalf of people with dementia and challenges health professionals to rethink what living with the diagnosis means. Where impaired cognition is suspected, a proper assessment of mental capacity is needed. Information should be tailored to the individual's needs and abilities.

Case example – ascertaining the wishes of a patient with dementia

B was in her early 90s with fluctuating capacity due to dementia. Doctors provisionally diagnosed her with bowel and liver cancer, but in order to confirm the diagnosis invasive investigations were required. Due to B's fluctuating capacity, doctors were unsure how to proceed. B had a good relationship with her family and her treating consultant suggested that family members attend her outpatient appointment with her. In the clinic, B seemed to accept the possible diagnosis of cancer, but she did not appear to want to make any decisions regarding further investigations and treatment. In a format agreed in the clinic, several close family members discussed the diagnosis and options with B. In these discussions, B communicated that she wanted to remain at home and not go into hospital. This was a consistent response, even when all the possible consequences of not going into hospital were explained to her. As a result, a treatment plan was implemented based on symptom management and B was cared for at home. She went on to enjoy a further 3 months of good quality life and died at home with her family.

Most people want to be involved in decisions affecting them but may want information at different stages rather than the same amount at the same pace. Discussion around treatment options should not be a once-and-for-all-time occurrence and information may need to be repeated. When people make clear that they want little information, it cannot be forced upon them but, in order for their consent to medical treatment to be valid, they need to know the core facts. This is discussed further in Chapters 3 and 4. Often it is relatives who ask for information to be withheld from older patients but the views that count are those of patients themselves. Due to stereotyping, however, health professionals often expect to encounter more difficulties with older people and so fail to offer as much information as they normally would. Studies indicate, for example, that doctors provide more information, are more supportive and more willing to share decision-making with younger rather than older patients[7]. This is unacceptable and the situation is exacerbated if older people appear unquestioning of the advice given.

Communication as an aid to planning and 'concordance'

Older people say that, when they are ill, they want to be included as part of the health care team and consulted more systematically than generally happens[8]. Some say they were unprepared for the information they later found in their medical notes, as they had not previously been told it. No one should have to find out what is wrong in this way. One of the criticisms made by patients and their relatives alike has been that the lack of candid information over a significant period left them quite unready to cope with the eventual severity of the patient's condition.

Everyone has the right to refuse treatment if he or she understands the implications. 'Concordance' is about patients understanding the advantages and disadvantages of specific treatment and why it is recommended for them. Concordance has been defined as 'shared decision-making and arriving at an agreement that respects the wishes and beliefs of the patient'[9]. Older people receive more prescriptions than other patients, with an increased risk of drug interactions and a higher rate of not completing a course of medication. Some evidence implies that older people 'are less ready for concordance'[10]. It is not necessarily the case that information is withheld from them but rather that they seem uninterested in knowing some of it. In a study of patients' understanding about warfarin as prophylaxis of thromboembolic conditions, for example, researchers found that patients were willing to take it without understanding why they should. Older people in the study had even less desire for information and were readier to follow doctors' recommendations without question. Although this might be seen as a positive indicator of the trust between patient and doctor, it is probably also a facet of an outdated culture in which older people were not offered much information. Patients' expectations are likely to be rather different in future as generations who have grown up with the current emphasis on autonomy reach old age. Best practice entails offering all patients at least a minimum of information about why a medication is recommended and its effects. Some patients who have suffered mental health problems, such as schizophrenia, throughout their lives but have successfully taken their medication for many years may become susceptible to a dementing illness in old age. This can adversely affect their ability to keep taking their medication and their overall health may suffer. Care providers need to be alert to this possibility.

In general, older people have higher risks of inappropriate prescriptions and of experiencing adverse reactions due to increased sensitivity to drugs' effects, reduced effectiveness of homoeostatic mechanisms and increased risk of idiosyncratic reactions[11]. Pharmacists can be helpful in backing up the information supplied by doctors and explaining to patients how their medication works, why they need it and whether they should refrain from self-medication. In residential care settings, older people often take responsibility for their own medication. The national minimum standards recognise the importance of this happening within a risk management framework[12]. Records must be kept of the current medication for each person. Apart from those which are self-administered, all other drugs should only be given by trained staff who understand the purpose of the medication. In hospitals and care homes, older people often complain that they are not told the reason for some medication nor given a choice about it. Reminding them what it is for is part of good practice and routine medication should be periodically reviewed, especially where a patient's condition may have changed or where multiple drugs are involved.

Communication with relatives

One of the common areas of misunderstanding concerns communication between health care staff and patients' relatives who often object to being excluded from discussions of a patient's care when the individual enters a hospital or nursing home. Most patients want their families to be kept informed and are quite capable themselves of passing on relevant information but they are also entitled to confidentiality[13]. Information about them should not be disclosed by carers without individuals' explicit agreement. Older people may assume that their spouse or close relatives will automatically be kept informed and this can, of course, happen if they make their wishes clear. Without such agreement, care providers cannot assume that patients want all their relatives to have confidential information. Relatives are not entitled to confidential information unless the patient has agreed or, if the person is incompetent to agree or refuse, it would be in that person's best interests.

Case example – respecting patients' confidentiality regarding relatives

Y was admitted to hospital for observation after a bad fall down some stairs. A widower, he was the centre of a close and caring family who were keen to be involved in all decisions affecting his care. Initially, he appeared happy with this. On admission, it was noted that he was a Jehovah's Witness and his signed declaration was lodged in his medical notes saying that he refused all blood products. When his family left, however, Y made clear that although he respected and sympathised with the JW religion, he was not committed to it in the way his children were and his late wife had been. He asked that his medical notes be amended to indicate his willingness to have blood products. He signed the notes, indicating that this was his current decision, overruling all previous decisions. This was witnessed by the doctor managing his care. Y specified that this information could not be shared with any members of his family, as he desperately wanted to avoid upsetting them or causing discord within the family. Good practice in this case involved having private discussions with the patient himself about his wishes rather than relying on what was said when his family was present. It also involved respecting his confidentiality even though this entailed the risk that the family might make decisions for him at some future date when he was unable to communicate, in the erroneous belief that he shared their values completely.

Another common communication problem arises when relatives insist that they alone be given information without it being shared with the patient. It is particularly worrying that such requests continue to proliferate, even in relation to older patients who are mentally competent and in cases where there might be potentially useful treatment options which the older person could be offered, if they were informed of them. As is emphasised throughout this report, it is important that the individual's own views are sought and respected.

Communication between people providing care

Poor communication between care providers is one of the most frequently cited causes of serious adverse events in health care. A breakdown in communication of data such as laboratory results can be due to a lack of clarity or absence of any prior agreement about who has responsibility for ensuring that other health professionals are kept informed. Reports from home visits by social workers or occupational therapists may also fail to be shared effectively. Among evidence gathered by the charity Help the Aged were examples of lack of co-ordination between health care staff or between health care providers and social care staff. In particular, communication appeared to break down most frequently when older patients were due to be discharged from hospital or transferred from one type of care to another[8]. Evidence of poor communication between health staff also occurred in hospital settings when health professionals providing specialised care had been informed about the patient's need for treatment but not given relevant information, such as the fact that the patient was blind or suffered from dementia. The National Institute for Health and Clinical Excellence has particularly highlighted the need for well-organised dementia care since evidence indicates that good organisation reduces disability[14]. Research also shows that 'much of the distress experienced by people with dementia and their families can be prevented when primary care works closely with geriatric nurse practitioners and community and voluntary services'[15]. Such working in partnership is the expected norm for various facets of caring for older people and requires good communication.

Multidisciplinary geriatric care

A randomised controlled trial was undertaken to assess the effectiveness of an interdisciplinary geriatric evaluation unit compared with the usual treatment (acute care followed by discharge to either home or long-term care facilities). Patients who fitted the eligibility criteria – over 64 years old who had a persistent medical, functional or psychological problem – were randomly allocated to the evaluation unit or the control group.

Among its stated goals, the evaluation unit aimed to increase the patient's level of functioning, improve diagnosis and treatment, achieve more appropriate placement, reduce the use of institutional services and generally increase the overall quality of care delivered to older patients. A multidisciplinary team involving doctors, specialist geriatric nurses, care assistants and a social worker ran the unit. There was also part-time input from a clinical psychologist, a dietician, a geriatric dentist, an audiologist, occupational therapists, physiotherapists and a public health nurse. The ratio of doctors and nurses to patients was equivalent to that on other intermediate care wards.

During the first year of follow-up, there was a significant difference in mortality between the two groups of older patients. In the evaluation unit, 23.8% died compared with 48.3% of the control group. More patients from the unit were discharged to their own homes (73%) compared with those in the control group (53.3%), who were more likely to be discharged to nursing homes. Morale among the unit patients was higher and they showed more improvement in functioning. They also spent less time in hospital acute care and had fewer readmissions to acute care[16].

Barriers to communication

An important first step in providing treatment or long-term care to older people is for staff to identify potential barriers to communication. Some are obvious such as the time pressure on health care staff and the fact that low-level hearing loss is common among older people. Even making a GP appointment via an automated telephone system can be challenging for people with hearing difficulties. Older people often come into contact with services at a time of stress and crisis when shock or anxiety reduce their ability to absorb information. Hearing aids and dentures may be removed or lost on admission to hospital or a care facility, which makes communication more difficult. Effective face-to-face communication can also be hampered by factors such as the difference in demographic characteristics and difference in expectations between the participants. Variations in class, race and ethnic background can affect how people communicate but age too can be a significant factor. These things need to be recognised and planned for so that avoidable barriers to good communication can be reduced.

Lack of training

Some health professionals and care providers have not been trained in effective communication or in identifying the particular needs of older people. Such training has been shown to effect significant improvements in interaction[3]. The Foundation for People with Learning Disabilities also points out that around half of the learning-disabled population have the same life expectancy as the general population but, even when young, many are looked after in care homes. Services and the training of care home staff rarely cater for their particular needs. These issues need to be addressed by residential homes providing care for this patient group.

Failure to see older patients as individuals with differing needs

Expecting patients to conform to a standard stereotype is often seen as a major issue for older people. Among the problems identified with end-of-life care by people involved in a Help the Aged study were lack of person-centred care, poor communication and inadequate information[8]. In fact, these problems are often interrelated. Older people consulted in the project were particularly concerned that, especially in a hospital setting, they were likely to be treated as a group rather than as individuals with differing needs and values. An example of complete lack of individualised care was a hospital patient being told not to make a fuss when she pointed out that the wrong name had been put above her bed. Very serious consequences can result from lack of communication among hospital staff about older patients' needs for help with eating and drinking. Trays of food and drink can be left beyond the reach of patients and then removed without discussion on the assumption that the individual is refusing food when staff are unaware that the patient needs help. This is discussed further in the section 'Raising difficult issues: elder abuse and neglect' (see page 23).

Case example – avoiding assumptions

H was admitted to hospital following a stroke. As he gradually recovered, he remained confused and it was assumed that he was unable to make even relatively small decisions such as what to wear. When H became agitated as he was dressed in the morning, it became obvious that he had very clear views about what he wanted to wear. Although H continued to have difficulty in communicating, he was increasingly able to indicate preferences and choices if he was given sufficient time and if carers used a basic sign language which acknowledged his difficulties. Small and very gradual improvements sometimes risk being overlooked which can lead to frustration and challenging behaviour by individuals who have suffered a serious cognitive impairment but who can still assert choices. In H's case, he remained severely impaired but continuing patient support helped him to extend the range of options upon which he could decide.

Concerns about being perceived as insensitive or racist

One of the barriers to effective communication with older patients can be health professionals' worry that if they speak frankly they may be seen as insensitive. Some patient groups fare particularly badly in this respect. A study in 2007, for example, highlighted the fact that many health professionals lacked confidence when dealing with ethnic minorities, and this could impinge on the way they provided care[17]. The study suggested that some health professionals felt that they did not know enough about different cultures and were worried about being perceived as racist. The researchers said that this created a 'disabling hesitancy' in health teams which could unintentionally contribute to ethnic disparities in health care. A thorough knowledge of different cultures is not essential but an open-minded approach is helpful when treating people from different cultural or ethnic backgrounds. Health professionals also need to be sensitive to other aspects of patients' lifestyle that might influence their choices, such as sexual orientation or past experience of mental health problems. A variation of the problem can arise in care homes which employ staff who have trained overseas. If patients and carers come from very different backgrounds, they can have differing expectations about how they should communicate with one another. Problems can be best avoided by advance recognition and discussion of the potential for misunderstandings. Older people, like any other patients, may also have racist attitudes and staff need to be trained to cope with the potential for racist abuse.

Elderspeak

Communication between health care providers and older patients can be undermined by the use of inappropriate styles of speech. These can either be overly controlling and so fail to reflect the autonomy of the individual addressed, or overly familiar using an inappropriate level of intimacy, which is known as 'elderspeak'. Professionals providing care to older people may inadvertently convey 'messages of dependence, incompetence and control to older adults by using elderspeak, a speech style similar to baby talk, that fails to communicate appropriate respect'[3]. This simplified communication is often intended to be reassuring rather than to have a negative effect. Some care providers become accustomed to using it in the absence of having had advice or training about communicating with older people. It is problematic because it represents a stereotyped response and implies that older people cannot cope with normal speech patterns. Typically, the rate of speech is slower, louder, more high pitched and uses more exaggerated intonation than normal adult speech. Repetition, simple vocabulary and simplified grammar also feature in it, along with diminutives and intimate terms of endearment, rather than individuals' names. Similar speech modifications are used with people with physical or mental disabilities. Elderspeak is more likely to occur in institutions than in similar interactions within the community. Although intended to be clear and sympathetic, this way of speech is both patronising and undermining to the individual hearing it, who often perceives it as demeaning. Because it implies less competence on the part of the listener, it is said that older people respond to it 'with lowered self-esteem, depression, withdrawal from social interactions and even dependent behaviour consistent with their own stereotypes of elderly individuals'[3]. One of the risks of elderspeak, therefore, is that it can strengthen dependency and bring about isolation and depression, which can lead to physical and cognitive decline[3].

Elderspeak may arise from habit or because professionals are advised to provide information in a manner 'appropriate' to the recipient. Older people living with various types of mental impairment, for example, can often make valid choices if these are effectively communicated to them. Emphasis on an appropriate manner of communication is intended to ensure that plain language is used instead of medical jargon and to ascertain whether the individual has hearing loss or needs language interpretation or signing.

Recording consultations and having an advocate present

Health professionals sometimes worry about patients tape recording consultations, seeing it as a sign of lack of trust or an intention to sue, particularly if done covertly. Patients' desire for a record of the meeting should be discussed in advance. People of any age often find it difficult to take in news that is bad, unexpected or very detailed. Recording can be particularly helpful for older people to remember accurately what was said but it also alters the nature of the conversation. Professionals may be less willing to speculate or explore areas of uncertainty. The World Health Organization (WHO) has highlighted how recordings or summaries of key consultations help cancer patients by improving their knowledge and recall without causing psychological problems[18]. WHO also makes the point that such tools 'must be used sensitively with patients whose prognosis is poor, and account must be taken of whether or not they wish to know the full facts' (Ref. [18], p. 26).

Alternatively, a relative or patient advocate taking notes can be helpful. Some patients need an intermediary if they have hearing or communication problems. Generally, it is good practice to involve relatives and it can help them understand the individual's needs but before any information is shared with family members, it is important to ascertain the patient's views. Sometimes an independent advocate with no emotional investment is the most appropriate person to support a patient. Independent advocacy services should be available for patients who want support in making decisions but it should be up to patients to choose if they want advocates to be involved. 'Advocacy' is defined as helping people to stand up for themselves and to be heard in situations when they feel they are not being taken seriously[19]. Advocates must be trained. It is not their job to tell patients what to do but rather to help individuals understand the choices and to represent their views. Patient advocacy services are provided by some charitable organisations and public service providers such as local authorities. Legally, patient advocates (even Independent Mental Capacity Advocates appointed under the Mental Capacity Act 2005 – see Chapter 4) have no formal decision-making powers but can facilitate good communication. This does not lessen the duty of health professionals to communicate effectively with patients themselves wherever possible. It is poor practice to talk solely to the advocate, excluding the patient. Conflict and misunderstandings can arise if roles are not properly defined and everyone involved in a decision needs to be aware of the scope and limits of advocates' powers.

Interpreters and facilities for the hard of hearing

Efforts should be made to meet the information needs of each patient, using interpreters, sign language communicators or advocates as appropriate. In 2007, a Healthcare Commission report[20] on dignity in the care for older people found that even when interpreters could be available, there was over-reliance in the NHS on asking relatives to interpret. This caused difficulties for patients presenting without family and those wanting to retain their privacy. Using relatives can lead to misinformation if patients are embarrassed about their relatives knowing all their symptoms, or if the relatives are embarrassed to translate some information. Older patients often want the support of relatives or carers but, particularly, if sensitive information is exchanged or some form of abuse against the individual is suspected, patient privacy needs to be a priority. Professionally qualified Public Service Interpreters should be used whenever possible as untrained, or poorly trained, interpreters can make mistakes or fail to provide an accurate verbatim account. Advance planning is required to achieve this. If nobody has informed the health team in advance that patients need language or signing assistance, the team may be uncertain how to respond to patients' needs or when to summon interpreters without causing offence[21].

Raising difficult issues: elder abuse and neglect

Care providers need good communication skills to broach some very sensitive and potentially distressing issues. Matters such as end-of-life care and where people would prefer to die are addressed in Chapter 8. Here we focus on the question of 'elder abuse'. This is 'a single or repeated act or lack of appropriate action occurring within any relationship where there is an expectation of trust, which causes harm or distress to an older person'[22]. It breaches Article 3 of the Human Rights Act 1998, which protects the right to be free from degrading treatment. Abuse involves the vulnerable sectors of society, including the sick, the old and people living with mental impairment. Older people experience more of the factors that make individuals vulnerable to abuse, such as social isolation, disability and illness. These combined with a general environment that fails to pay attention to individuals' dignity creates the potential for abuse.

Although often described as a hidden problem[23], awareness of elder abuse has significantly risen over recent years through a series of policy developments, campaigns and media coverage. Estimates vary of how many older people suffer abuse, due to difficulties in identifying it, imprecision about what the term covers and the fact that adults with cognitive impairments are often excluded from research. The true extent of the problem is difficult to identify. In 2007, a UK prevalence study[24] concluded that around 342,400 or 1 in 25 older people experienced abuse. Neglect was found to be the most prominent form of mistreatment, followed by financial, physical and psychological abuse. Neglect featured particularly in the mistreatment of women over the age of 85 and the main perpetrators were partners (who may themselves be elderly) and other relatives. Some abuse stems from relatives becoming unable to cope and arrangements need to be made to ensure the safety of the older person. Respite care can be an interim solution until the situation can be reassessed.

Another report estimated that about a third of abusers were paid workers[22]. In those cases, abuse is more likely where paid helpers work on their own for long periods, without supervision or peer review. Teams which lack effective leadership can also be prone to team members tolerating poor practice and not speaking out against it. Almost a quarter of the reports of abuse on the Action on Elder Abuse helpline relate to care homes, where less than 5% of the older population live, and only 5% relate to care in hospital[22]. This low figure may well reflect a widespread lack of training in knowing how to recognise and address signs of abuse and neglect. In 2007, for example, a poll of nurses found that more than half would not report evidence of abuse of an elderly person in their care[24]. Lack of training in how to deal with it was one reason but also fear of confrontation or of upsetting the victim also inhibited nurses from speaking out. Sometimes they feared that they might have misinterpreted what was going on. In residential and inpatient settings, abuse or neglect can arise through inattention or bad communication. Health professionals particularly need to be alert to:

- neglect, including removing aids such as spectacles, hearing aids, false teeth or a call bell or leaving these things out of patients' reach. Spectacles and hearing aids may also be lost as patients are moved around and staff may fail to look for them;
- lack of assistance with feeding, or food and drink left out of reach, which can result in serious malnutrition or dehydration and mental confusion;
- health problems, including hearing and visual problems, left uncorrected;
- poor hygiene and inadequate levels of personal care which can lead to infection and bedsores;
- over-medication or sedation of patients primarily to make their care easier.

The Parliamentary Human Rights Committee drew attention to a typical tragic case involving the neglect of a hospital patient who was not helped to eat and drink despite her physical inability to feed herself. Visitors who wanted to help her were discouraged from staying during meal times. Eventually the patient 'appeared to be slowly starving to death'[26]. In cases such as this, it is clear that carers have a duty to address immediately all the factors contributing to the patient's condition. (More detailed information on the issue of the abuse of older people is flagged up in the section at the end of the chapter on resources and other sources of advice.)

Clearly, it is a serious problem which health professionals need to know how to recognise. Some forms of deliberate abuse are hard to identify unless patients disclose information. Frail older people with mobility problems are susceptible to accidental injuries but any evidence of non-accidental injury needs to be investigated, including repeated fractures, bruises or burns on less-exposed parts of the body. Often, however, there are no obvious external signs. It is estimated that only a fraction of older people suffering abuse feature in adult protection procedures. It is essential that care providers know how to engage with such procedures. All local authorities and most trusts have a Safeguarding Adults policy. Health and social care professionals need to be aware of such local arrangements and how to take action if abuse is suspected. They cannot promise confidentiality if other people may also be at risk and a balance needs to be found between respecting the wishes of the victim – who may not want disclosure – and ensuring that abuse is tackled effectively. Prompt arrangements need to be made to ensure the older person's safety. Details of the abuse should be documented and reported to a line manager who can pursue the matter with the local Safeguarding Adults Co-ordinator. Some types of suspected abuse, such as financial or emotional exploitation, can be difficult to identify but professionals can make clear their willingness to listen to patients with such concerns. Providing support can be difficult if the older person is unwilling to allow disclosure and this is discussed further in Chapter 5 on confidentiality.

Summary of chapter

- *Effective communication with older people takes time, training and thought.*
- *Like everyone else, older people have rights to make their own decisions.*
- *Relevant information about the options should be offered in a way they can understand.*
- *Good communication is also about listening and attempting to find out what precisely the recipient needs to know.*
- *Discussing the suspected abuse of older people is as difficult and fraught an issue as dealing with suspected child abuse or domestic violence.*
- *Where older people seem to be in danger, action needs to be taken in line with local policies on Safeguarding Adults and guidance from professional bodies, such as the GMC which regulates doctors. This topic is followed up in Chapter 5.*

References

1. Alzheimer's Society (2007). *Home from Home: A Report Highlighting Opportunities for Improving Standards of Dementia Care in Care Homes.* Alzheimer's Society, London.
2. Commission for Social Care Inspection (2008). *See Me, Not Just the Dementia: Understanding People's Experience of Living in a Care Home.* CSCI, London.
3. Williams K, Kemper S, Hummert ML (2004). Enhancing communication with older adults: overcoming elderspeak. *J Gerontol Nurs* **30(10):** 17–25.
4. General Medical Council (2008). *Consent: Patients and Doctors Making Decisions Together.* GMC, London, p. 11.
5. Payne SA (2002). Balancing information needs: dilemmas in producing patient information leaflets. *Health Informatics J* **8:** 174–9.
6. The Scottish Dementia Working Group is an independent group run by people with dementia.
7. See, for example, Adelman RD, Greene MG, Charon R (1991). Issues in the physician–elderly patient interaction. *Aging and Soc* **2:** 127–48.

8. Clarke A, Seymour J, Welton M, Sanders C, Gott M (2006). *Listening to Older People: Opening the Door for Older People to Explore End-of-Life Issues.* Help the Aged, London.

9. Jones G (2003). Prescribing and taking medicines: concordance is a fine theory but is mostly not being practiced. *Br Med J* **327:** 819–20.

10. Engova D, Duggan C, MacCallum P, et al. (2002). Patients' understanding and perceptions of treatment as determinants of adherence to warfarin treatment. *Int J Pharm Pract* **10(suppl):** R69.

11. British Medical Association (2007). *Evidence-Based Prescribing.* BMA, London.

12. Department of Health (2002). *Care Homes for Older People. National Minimum Standards. Care Home Regulations: Third Edition.* The Stationery Office Ltd, London, p. 9.

13. This is discussed in detail in Chapter 5 on confidentiality.

14. The National Institute for Health and Clinical Excellence and the Social Care Institute for Excellence (2006). *Dementia: The NICE-SCIE Guideline on Supporting People with Dementia and Their Carers in Health and Social Care.* The British Psychological Society, Leicester.

15. Downs M, Bowers B (2008). Caring for people with dementia. *Br Med J* **336:** 225–6.

16. Rubenstein L, Josephson K, Wieland GD, et al. (1984). Effectiveness of a geriatric evaluation unit. *N Engl J Med* **311:** 1664–70.

17. Kai J, Beavan J, Faull C, Dodson L, Gill P, et al. (2007). Professional uncertainty and disempowerment responding to ethnic diversity in health care: a qualitative study. *PLoS Med* 4(11): e323. Public Library of Science, Cambridge.

18. World Health Organization Europe. Davies R, Higginson IJ (eds) (2004). *Better Palliative Care for Older People.* WHO, Copenhagen.

19. Nancy K (2005). *The Mind Guide to Advocacy.* Mind, London.

20. Healthcare Commission (2007). *Caring for Dignity: A National Report on Dignity in Care for Older People While in Hospital.* Commission for Healthcare Audit and Inspection, London.

21. Training programmes such as the PROCEED programme (Professionals Responding to Cancer and Ethnic Diversity) aim to develop generic skills to help professionals respond appropriately to patients' needs for language interpretation.

22. Action on Elder Abuse (2004). *Hidden Voices: Older People's Experience of Abuse. An Analysis of Calls to the Action on Elder Abuse Helpline.* Help the Aged, London.

23. House of Commons Health Committee (2004). *Elder Abuse Second Report of Session 2003–04. Volume 1.* The Stationery Office Ltd, London, paras 3 and 15.

24. O'Keeffe M, Hills A, Doyle M, et al. (2007). *UK Study of Abuse and Neglect of Older People Prevalence Study Report.* King's College London and National Centre for Social Research, London.

25. Ward L. Nurses loth to report abuse of the elderly. *The Guardian* 29 August, 2007.

26. House of Lords, House of Commons, Joint Committee on Human Rights (2007). *The Human Rights of Older People in Healthcare, Eighteenth Report of Session 2006–07. Volume 2 – Oral and Written Evidence.* The Stationery Office, London, Ev 104, para 1 (c).

Further resources

Northern Ireland Department of Health, Social Services and Public Safety (2006). *Safeguarding Vulnerable Adults: Regional Adult Protection Policy and Procedural Guidance.* DHSSPS, Belfast.

The British Medical Association (2004). *Communication Education Skills for Doctors: An Update.* BMA, London.

The Department of Health (2000). *No Secrets: Guidance on Developing and Implementing Multi-agency Policies and Procedures to Protect Vulnerable Adults from Abuse.* DH, London.

The National Assembly for Wales (2000). *In Safe Hands: Implementing Adult Protection Procedures in Wales.* The National Assembly for Wales, Cardiff.

The Scottish Government (2008). *Code of Practice for Part 1 of the Adult Support and Protection (Scotland) Act 2007.* The Scottish Government, Edinburgh.

Chapter 3 **Ethical issues regarding consent and refusal**

The right to choice in health care

Providing patients with information about care and treatment options is an important way of respecting their autonomy. The regulatory body for medicine, the General Medical Council (GMC), particularly emphasises that patients and doctors should make decisions together[1]. Discriminating attitudes mean that some procedures are not offered to older people who could benefit from them, although younger people with similar conditions would be told about them. Difficult choices need to be made if the treatment carries high risks. It is sometimes assumed that the risks of surgery, for example, outweigh the benefits for people in the later years of life but patients themselves should be allowed to make those difficult choices. They should have opportunities to weigh up the advantages and disadvantages, if there is a likelihood of benefit. When the risks and benefits of treatment are not clear-cut, individuals' preferences are even more important. Offering choices to older patients is not 'an optional extra' and even if they have declined a treatment previously, they may want to reconsider if circumstances change.

Case example – keeping open the choice about surgery

M had long suffered from arthritis and pain in her hip but had refused a hip replacement. When the pain became worse, her GP recommended that she reconsider surgery. Two of M's relatives who had hip replacements had suffered hip dislocations afterwards, which left them less mobile than before. M assumed that the alleged benefits were overblown and feared that surgery might leave her worse off. M's specialist agreed that there was a small risk that M could be left less mobile but thought that surgery could provide a significant advantage for her. He explained that support and equipment would be provided by a community care team after surgery but strict rules needed

---

The Ethics of Caring for Older People 2nd Edition. By British Medical Association. Published 2009 by Blackwell Publishing Limited, ISBN: 9781405176279.

to be followed to avoid damaging the new hip. In the past, he said, patients' failure to achieve an improvement had often been due to their not following carefully enough the recommended post-operative regime. The specialist suggested that he and M look again at the pros and cons and identify her precise worries about the surgery, which he thought could be life changing. He also discussed with M the likely progression of her condition if no action was taken. Many of M's objections concerned the degree of genuine improvement she could expect and practical worries about how she would cope in the rehabilitation period. She decided to accept surgery once she felt that her anxieties had been taken seriously.

The right to opportunities for choice in other types of care

In any scenario in which care is provided for older people, they should have an input into decisions affecting them. Outside the health care situation, choice should be promoted wherever possible in the provision of broader care activities. These include the provision of meals and appropriate nutrition to take account of individuals' preferences and their religious or cultural requirements. Also help with activities such as washing, bathing and toileting should reflect individual choice as much as possible. The National Service Framework for Older People attempts to counter age discrimination by highlighting the need to view older people as active participants in, rather than the subjects of, the care-providing process[2]. This aim to promote active participation in decision-making is as important in choices such as where people live as it is in medical treatment decisions.

Case example – participation in care choices

C experienced intermittent confusion and lapses of memory. He sometimes found himself at a busy junction near his residential care home, without being able to recall how he got there. Although this worried him, he was even more worried that arrangements would be made to transfer him to a more restrictive environment without consulting him. In fact, his son had already begun arrangements for C to move to an enclosed facility in which residents were unable to leave the building. The care team pointed out that C first needed a proper psychiatric assessment to clarify the level of care he needed and whether his current arrangements could be adapted. Proposals for change needed to be discussed with C when he was most lucid rather than being decided behind his back. Although confused at times, C's dementia was mild. He was aware that he needed to protect his own safety and was willing to agree to compromises in order to stay in his familiar setting. It was important for him not to be treated as mentally incompetent when he could make valid choices and, with support, manage his own affairs.

Explicit and implied consent to treatment

Adults are presumed to have the mental capacity to accept or refuse medical treatment, irrespective of their age or physical condition, unless evidence indicates the contrary. In cases of doubt about mental capacity, a formal assessment is required. If they are competent, individuals' agreement is required for examination or treatment, except in emergencies or where compulsory treatment is given under mental health legislation. Seeking consent involves offering information about options but in many situations, consent is implied by patients' co-operation and may not be explicitly stated. They tacitly indicate agreement by offering an arm for blood pressure to be taken or swallowing the pills offered to them. Implicit consent is so common in routine encounters that care professionals can become blasé and take it for granted that patients want a treatment, without necessarily discussing it fully. Time pressures can also tempt staff to cut corners and not provide proper explanations. This is poor practice. Consent is only implied if individuals understand in general terms what they are consenting to. Otherwise, there is no consent at all. Acquiescence is not 'consent' if people do not know what a treatment or medication entails or that they have an option of refusing. Even if they appear unquestioning, competent patients have the right to be properly informed.

Providing accurate information

The importance of providing people with sufficient information to enable them to make an informed choice is highlighted in Chapter 2. Without relevant information about healthcare options, a person's consent or refusal could be invalid. What constitutes 'sufficient' information varies with what the individual wants to know, the complexity of the procedure, its risks and any other serious implications. Most people want more than just a list of alternatives and need advice about which treatment is likely to be the most appropriate for their individual circumstances. Questions should be answered truthfully and health professionals should be prepared to share uncertainty with patients, where appropriate. As well as information about their condition, options for treatment, information about aftercare and risks and benefits, patients need to know about the implications of doing nothing. They may also want to know where treatment will be given, whether it involves a stay in hospital and how long recovery will take. Clear patient information leaflets can be useful but do not replace discussion. If patients are very ill, hard of hearing or have difficulty communicating, there can be a temptation to discuss care primarily with relatives. In extreme cases, this may be the only option but should not be the first resort.

Case example – offering information

F was admitted to hospital in an acute confusional state with a serious chest infection. She was suffering from consolidation of the lower lobe of her right lung and was delirious. Her family insisted on knowing her diagnosis which they understood could either be pneumonia or lung cancer. Tests showed that she had a malignant bronchial tumour but that her mental confusion was unrelated to the cancer. It was due to an infection which quickly improved with antibiotics. As F regained mental capacity, the oncologist went to discuss her diagnosis with her, including options for treatment and palliative care, but found that the family had misled F into believing that she had had pneumonia, with no need for further treatment. Her relatives were adamant that F should not be told about the cancer. Having looked on the Internet at the success rates for treatment of lung cancer, they felt it was unlikely to improve her condition. The health team were reluctant to contradict the family but could not tell F lies about her diagnosis. They needed sensitively to probe her own wishes about how much information she wanted and discuss palliative care treatment, rather than allowing the family to pre-empt that. In discussion, it became clear that F wanted to discuss her diagnosis and treatment options, having suspected that her family were hiding things. She emphasised that the choices should be hers and that she definitely wanted to have palliative care arranged as soon as possible.

It is not uncommon for relatives to insist that an older person not be told about a diagnosis of cancer but it is important that patients' own views are heard, if they are competent and willing to know.

Refusing information

In some cases, patients do not want full information but they should be aware of the basic options. Without some core information, they are unable to make valid choices. Most people manage to deal with difficult news despite their anxieties, if they are given support and if the choices are explained to them in a sensitive manner. The GMC has advice about situations in which patients decline information[1]. It says that doctors should first explain to patients why it is important for them to understand the options. If, after discussion, the patient refuses to know the details, that decision should be respected but doctors must still provide enough basic information for the patient to give valid consent to the proposed treatment or investigation. It is sometimes suggested that patients refusing information should be asked to sign a waiver, if the implications of not receiving information could be serious. A waiver simply documents that information was offered. Many health professionals are not keen on the use of a waiver, as its main purpose is to prevent patients or relatives later complaining that the care providers were negligent in not giving information. Waivers are often seen as symptomatic of defensive medicine and lack of trust between doctor and patient.

Recording consent and refusal

Consent to treatment may be given orally, in writing or by other means such as signing by patients who are deaf. Refusal can be expressed in the same way by patients who understand the implications. A written consent form, often seen as evidence of consent, simply shows that some discussion has taken place. Health professionals worry about not having a signature on a consent form if, for example, older patients whose sight is severely impaired cannot read and sign it. A witnessed verbal agreement by blind patients should be sufficient since the validity of consent depends on the quality of the information given and whether the recipient understands it. Patients' signed consent or refusal may be invalid if crucial information is withheld from them when the choice is made. In some instances, a patient advocate may need to provide support to a patient making a treatment decision or a proxy decision-maker may be involved in giving consent. Such situations are discussed in Chapter 4. In many cases, there is no specific need for consent to be written, but if complex or risky procedures are proposed, it is advisable. Written consent is also usual for surgery, for participation in medical research and for interventions intended primarily to benefit somebody else other than the person undergoing it, such as DNA testing to help a family member. Consent forms are also a legal requirement under certain parts of mental health legislation[3]. Refusal of treatment should be documented if it has serious or life-threatening implications. Chapter 7 covers the advisability of a written record when patients' refusal of treatment is likely to result in premature death.

Consent to participate in research

Older people should have opportunities to participate in medical or social research. Often they are keen to do so, and not just for altruistic reasons. Participation in qualitative research has the potential to increase the understanding of their experience and perspectives. Such research can also provide a sense of satisfaction and being listened to, but it also has the potential for distress if sensitive issues are explored. Participation in some drug trials provides early access to promising new therapies, but not all participants can expect to benefit, as they may be randomised to a placebo or a standard product. Many drug trials provide regular health monitoring in order to exclude other health risks which would skew the results and this can be beneficial to participants. All medical research must be subject to ethical scrutiny and participants need to know the risks, side effects and implications for their care. When older people will not benefit personally from the research or when more than minimal risk is involved, it is crucial that they understand that. They should also feel able to give consent or refusal without any pressure being exerted. Although many older people are willing to participate in research, society's anxiety about exploiting their vulnerability can make ethics committees reluctant to authorise it. Age barriers are also imposed on medical research due to the increased likelihood of co-morbidities, but narrow selection criteria can unfairly disadvantage older people by imposing arbitrary age restrictions. For example, one review[4] of 225 research proposals found that 85 studies had an inappropriate age restriction. When approached, however, older people are more likely to consider participation in clinical trials than younger adults[5].

In terms of social research, society can be overprotective in its reluctance to seek older people's views on sensitive topics, such as bereavement, ageing and the end of life. This can make them feel marginalised and frustrated about being excluded from discussion of issues that affect them more than other groups. One study[6] looked, for example, at the way research about what constitutes a 'good death' was hampered by a reluctance to talk to people facing death, in case it upset them. Some people in that situation are keen to discuss their fears and feelings, especially if it helps others. Automatically excluding older people from such projects negates their right to make their own choices.

Older people who have impaired mental capacity can also be involved in research with safeguards. (These are set out in Chapter 4.) The research should either be in their interests or not contrary to their interests and must be scrutinised by an ethics committee. It must also potentially benefit people in the same category. Such research is only ethical if it is not possible to carry it out involving competent people. Research into dementia care, for example, needs to involve people affected by the condition. Some research, such as that using anonymised data, does not require consent, regardless of whether or not the individual has mental capacity.

Assessing capacity to consent or refuse

In order to choose in a valid way, people must have the mental capacity to understand what the choice entails, at the time the decision is made. All adults are assumed to have this ability unless there is evidence to the contrary. The British Medical Association and the Law Society have jointly issued a book for doctors and lawyers, setting out the detailed procedures for assessing a person's mental capacity[7].

Capacity can be temporarily affected by dehydration, infection, medication or fatigue, but assumptions about impairment cannot be based on age alone or frailty. Nor can they be based on hearing, sight or speech impediments. Efforts must be made to talk to people when they are at their best and treatable physical problems which could affect their cognitive functioning must be addressed. A wide spectrum of ability is found in people deemed to have impaired competence, including those living with dementia or with learning disabilities. It is important, therefore, to see each person as an individual. Disease or other factors can result in temporary, fluctuating or enduring incapacity.

Case example – assessing mental capacity

O's relatives thought that she was sliding into dementia when she appeared confused, acted out of character, dressed strangely, was uninhibitedly rude and gave bizarre answers to questions. Her GP was asked to carry out an assessment of her mental capacity in anticipation of O being admitted to a specialist care home. The GP had known O for years and was familiar with her reluctance to admit to health problems or ask for help. After talking to O, she concluded that deafness was causing O to answer bizarrely as she often misheard the question. Macular degeneration affecting her eyesight caused O to make wildly inappropriate choices of clothing, ignore friends and greet strangers. O also experienced some mental confusion, caused by dehydration as O's fear of incontinence made her reluctant to take liquids. Antibiotics rectified her confusion but her failing eyesight meant that O needed a higher level of care than could be provided in her home. Rather than being diagnosed with dementia, she was assessed as being partially sighted and agreed to moving to a general care home, close to her relatives.

Odd choices or behavioural or cultural differences are not indicators of impaired cognition. The law establishes that different levels of understanding are essential for different types of decision. (This is discussed more in Chapter 4 and also in the joint BMA and Law Society's publication.) In crude terms, the graver the implications of a particular choice, the more important it is that individuals understand what they are letting themselves in for. Decisions which appear rash or unconventional are not indicators of impaired capacity but can raise questions about whether a formal assessment is needed.

Case example – assessing mental capacity

P was admitted to a residential care home after the death of his son, his last surviving relative. Other residents complained about P's behaviour. He failed to observe social conventions, wandered into other people's rooms uninvited and helped himself to their fruit. He was extremely talkative and carried on lengthy conversations with himself late at night. An assessment of P's mental state was requested. When his history was unravelled, it appeared that P and his wife came to the United Kingdom to join their son but P's wife had died from breast cancer and his son was later killed in a traffic accident, leaving P without any family or a social network. His problems were social isolation, loneliness and unfamiliarity with English social norms. Dropping in on neighbours and sharing food was common in the community in which he had spent his life. P was assessed as mentally competent and in need of advice about expectations in the care home. He needed to be included in social activities and have opportunities to meet other compatriots.

Practicalities of assessing mental capacity

Usually, it is self-evident whether or not a person has sufficient mental capacity to make a particular decision. Where doubts arise, the GP is often best placed to give a view, especially if there has been close contact and the patient feels relaxed with a familiar doctor. Assessment cannot be rushed. It is important that the assessing doctor has background information, about both the patient's medical history and the decision for which the patient is being assessed. Judging whether an individual has the mental capacity to make a valid will, for example, is a different matter to assessing whether that person can choose between medical treatment options or contract to sell a house. Carers and people emotionally close to the patient can often add supplementary information. Various facets of individuals' appearance and behaviour need to be taken into account and can indicate, for example, whether they have a mood disorder, such as depression or anxiety, or cognitive impairment. Delusions and other abnormalities of thought need to be assessed. The flow of patients' speech and whether their conversation moves in a disordered way between different topics can also indicate abnormal thought processes. Damage to the brain's language areas following a stroke can make direct verbal communication impossible with some patients. Many older people also have problems with their long-term memory. This is not necessarily any indication of reduced mental capacity but inability to remember information long enough to make a decision would invalidate it.

In cases of persisting doubt and when the decision has potentially serious consequences, it is advisable to organise a formal assessment by a psychiatrist or psychologist. If patients have borderline or fluctuating capacity, it can be particularly difficult to assess whether they can make valid decisions at a specific time. On some occasions, they probably can and at other times, the validity of their choice is questionable. The fact that people have a mental disorder, learning disability or some other impairment does not necessarily prevent them from making valid choices and so again, an individualised approach is essential. If people appear to lack capacity, it is normally possible to assess their abilities through a conversation, but if they refuse assessment, it cannot proceed unless required by a court. After a stroke, for example, some patients who can communicate find it difficult to organise their thoughts and may strongly object to being asked even apparently innocuous questions. If it is clear that a person lacks mental capacity to give valid consent or refusal, decisions on his or her behalf are governed by the Mental Capacity Act 2005 in England and Wales, by the Adults With Incapacity Act 2000 in Scotland and by common law in Northern Ireland. (These are discussed in Chapter 4.)

Assessment criteria in relation to choosing medical treatment

A formal assessment includes deciding whether the individual can:
- *understand in simple language what the treatment is, its purpose and nature and why it is being proposed;*
- *understand its principal benefits, risks and alternatives;*
- *understand in broad terms what will be the consequences of not receiving the proposed treatment;*
- *retain the information long enough to make a decision.*

Where the assessment concludes that the individual lacks capacity to make the decision in question at that particular time, it is irrelevant whether the incapacity is temporary or permanent. If capacity fluctuates, or is temporary, and the decision can realistically be put off, it should be deferred until the person is better able to deal with it. Basically, everything practicable should be done to help people make their own decisions.

'Best interests' or 'benefit'

If people lack mental capacity to make a particular choice, any decision on their behalf must be based on their 'best interests' in England, Wales and Northern Ireland or, in Scotland, what would 'benefit' them. Assessing where their best interests lie, or what would provide a benefit, means looking at several factors including the circumstances of the case and the individual's known past wishes, which may be recorded in a written statement or 'living will' (see Chapter 7). A proxy decision-maker must take into account whether the person is likely to regain capacity and, if so, whether decisions can reasonably be postponed until that time. A crucial part of deciding what is in another person's best interests or to his or her benefit involves discussion with those close to the individual, including family, friends or carers and anyone legally nominated to act as a proxy decision-maker. (More information about talking to such people is given in Chapters 2 and 4.)

Proxy consent

Recent legislation in England, Wales and Scotland concerning the care and treatment of adults who lack capacity has bought in powers to appoint proxy decision-makers. Codes of Practice supporting the legislation provide detailed information about the powers and responsibilities of these proxy decision-makers and address issues such as confidentiality and disclosure of information. The Mental Capacity Act in England and Wales also introduced a statutory advocacy service for when serious decisions need to be made on behalf of particularly vulnerable adults. These legal aspects, which are discussed in more detail in Chapter 4, draw heavily on established best practice.

Summary of chapter

- *Older people – like all other patients – need to be approached as individuals when they are offered information and choices in a health care setting.*
- *Care providers must keep an open mind and not have pre-existing assumptions about older people's abilities or needs.*

- *When patients already have a diagnosis of mental impairment, that should not be interpreted as necessarily implying that they cannot make valid choices.*
- *There is an ethical obligation to help people make their own choices to the degree that they are able and to maximise their abilities by carrying out assessments in familiar premises and helping them choose at times when they are likely to be most lucid.*

References

1. General Medical Council (2008). *Consent: Patients and Doctors Making Decisions Together*. GMC, London.
2. Department of Health (2001). *National Service Framework for Older People*. DH, London.
3. Mental Health Act 1983. Mental Health (Care and Treatment) (Scotland) Act 2003. Mental Health (Northern Ireland) Order 1986.
4. Bayer A, Tad W (2000). Unjustified exclusion of elderly people from studies submitted to research ethics committee for approval: descriptive study. *Br Med J* **321:** 992–3.
5. McMurdo MET, Witham MD, Gillespie N (2005). Including older people in clinical research. *Br Med J* **331:** 1036–7.
6. Kendall M, Harris F, Boyd K, Sheikl A, et al. (2007). Key challenges and ways forward in researching the 'good death'. *Br Med J* **334:** 521–4.
7. British Medical Association and The Law Society (2004). *Assessment of Mental Capacity: Guidance for Doctors and Lawyers: Second Edition*. BMJ Books, London. Third edition due 2009.

Further resources

British Medical Association (2008). *Consent Tool Kit: Fourth Edition*. BMA, London.

British Medical Association and The Law Society (2004). *Assessment of Mental Capacity: Guidance for Doctors and Lawyers: Second Edition*. BMJ Books, London. Third edition due 2009.

General Medical Council (2008). *Consent: Patients and Doctors Making Decisions Together*. GMC, London.

The Health Departments for England, Wales, Scotland and Northern Ireland publish guidance on consent. Contact details for each of the Departments are provided in 'Useful Organisations', at the end of this guidance.

Chapter 4 **Legal issues regarding consent and refusal**

The legislation covered here includes:
- the common law (across the United Kingdom);
- the Mental Capacity Act 2005 (in England and Wales);
- Adults with Incapacity (Scotland) Act 2000 (in Scotland);
- Human Rights Act 1998 (across the United Kingdom).

Older people with mental capacity

The common law on consent to examination, treatment and research

The legal rules on patient consent and refusal are established by common law and are similar to the ethical rules, set out in Chapter 3. Before examining or treating patients, health professionals must ensure that the patient knows what is involved and gives consent. Emergency situations are an exception to this rule, as are cases where compulsory treatment is authorised by mental health legislation. The law assumes that all adults have the mental capacity to make decisions, unless the contrary can be demonstrated. This is relevant to the care of older people, since institutional pressures, communication difficulties or negative stereotyping can lead to unfounded assumptions about their abilities. The law is clear that the onus to demonstrate that an adult lacks mental capacity is on those who believe that to be the case. Care providers have both moral and legal duties to take all reasonable steps to enable people to decide for themselves, whenever they can.

For consent or refusal to be legally valid, individuals must:
- have a general understanding of the decision to be made and why they need to make it;
- have a general understanding of the likely consequences of making or not making it;
- be able to understand, retain, use and weigh up relevant information;
- be acting voluntarily and free from pressure;
- be aware that they have options to consent or refuse.

The Ethics of Caring for Older People 2nd Edition. By British Medical Association. Published 2009 by Blackwell Publishing Limited, ISBN 9781405176279.

In many instances, there is no legal requirement to obtain written consent but for very serious or risky interventions, or for medical research, it is advisable[1]. (The use of anonymised aggregated data for research does not require consent.) A consent form documents that some discussion about the procedure or investigation has taken place. The quality and accuracy of the information given to the individual are paramount considerations in deciding whether a competent adult's decision is legally valid or not. If individuals refuse to have even core information about their condition or its recommended treatment, the validity of their subsequent decisions about their care may be in doubt (see Chapter 3).

Refusal of treatment by competent adults

Consent and refusal are often part of a continuing process rather than one-off decisions. As long as they are mentally competent, individuals have the option of changing their minds. Legally, they can refuse most treatments (except some mental health assessments and care) at the time it is proposed or in advance (see Chapter 7). Competent adults have legal rights to refuse treatment even when that will result in their death. Jehovah's Witnesses, for example, can refuse blood products essential for their survival. Where the consequences of refusal are grave, it is important that patients understand this. Health professionals must respect a refusal of treatment if the patient is competent, properly informed and is not coerced.

Case example – treatment refusal

The fact that D spent several years in a care home prolonged her life significantly but she greatly missed her home and garden. Her health problems were well managed by medication and oxygen to assist her breathing. D was a widow whose circle of relatives diminished year by year. When D received news of her sister's death, she seemed to make up her mind to die and became unwilling to accept her medication or to eat. She asked for the oxygen cylinders to be removed from her room and spent more time in bed. Staff asked for her to be assessed by the community mental health team as they thought she might be suffering from depression or be confused due to her reduced intake of liquids. D was judged to be competent and fully aware of the outcome of her decisions. Although sad, she was not judged to be suffering from depression. Her life was drawing to a close at a pace she dictated. Food continued to be offered but she only accepted sips of water and made it clear that she did not want artificial feeding, even if she became unconscious. The staff took turns in sitting with her during the final days. D seemed content with this and died soon after.

Impaired capacity to consent to or refuse treatment

When people are suspected of having impaired mental capacity, an assessment needs to take place (see Chapter 3). If individuals lack the ability to make a specific decision, they should still be involved as far as possible in the decision-making process but the law prescribes how the decision is to be made. In England and Wales, the Mental Capacity Act specifies the criteria for decision-making. In Scotland, the Adults with Incapacity Act fulfils the same function. In Northern Ireland, such decisions are governed by common law. Despite regional variations, there are common principles throughout the United Kingdom and these are set out below. In England and Wales, the Mental Capacity Act and its Code of Practice[2] provide detailed advice. Health professionals, care providers and others acting in a professional capacity or for remuneration have a legal obligation to take account of the Code when making decisions on behalf of someone who is incapacitated. In Scotland, the Adults with Incapacity (Scotland) Act also has a Code of Practice[3] which specifies that anyone carrying out functions under the Act must apply the general principles explained in the Code. The Code's aim is to provide flexibility to tailor interventions to fit the needs of individual cases.

General principles for action on behalf of incapacitated adults

- Any decision must be in the 'best interests' of the incapacitated adult or must 'benefit' that person. (The Mental Capacity Act and the common law in Northern Ireland refer to 'best interests'; the Adults With Incapacity (Scotland) Act talks about 'benefit' – see below.)
- Any intervention should be the least restrictive option in relation to the freedom of the incapacitated person.
- Interventions should take account of the past and present known wishes of the adult.
- Incapacitated adults should be encouraged to exercise as much as possible their own decision-making abilities.
- Consultation should include relevant people close to the incapacitated person.

'Best interests' and 'benefit'

In England, Wales and Northern Ireland, the law is based on the notion of 'best interests', whereas in Scotland it is based on 'benefit'. In either case, it is not simply a matter of making decisions solely about maximising clinical improvement but also reflecting less tangible benefits, such as respecting patients' values. Some people, for example, have made it clear in the past that they would not want life-prolonging treatment if there was no hope of them regaining their mental abilities. For them, life-prolonging treatment is not a benefit nor in their best interests as it would not reflect their known wishes. An objective assessment has to be made of what would be in individuals' overall best interests, bearing in mind their previous wishes. Relatives can often indicate whether the incapacitated person would have wanted a particular treatment in the situation which has arisen.

Guide to identifying 'best interests'

The Mental Capacity Act identifies factors that must be taken into account when making a best interests assessment. These reflect general good practice across the United Kingdom and can be summarised as:

- *doing whatever is practical to encourage and help the person to participate in making the decision;*
- *identifying things that the person would take into account if acting for him- or herself;*
- *reflecting the person's known wishes and any statement made before capacity was lost;*
- *identifying the values that would be likely to influence the decision if the patient had capacity;*
- *avoiding assumptions about a person's best interests based on the person's age, appearance, condition or behaviour;*
- *considering whether the person is likely to regain capacity;*
- *consulting other people, where practical, for their views about the person's best interests[2].*

Fluctuating capacity

Some individuals do not completely lose their mental capacity but their abilities fluctuate. They need to continue to be involved, as much as they can be, in the decisions affecting them. Non-urgent decisions may be postponed until people are at their most lucid. Sensitive and sometimes repeated assessments of the individual's capacity and needs are required. Otherwise, such people may be assumed to be permanently mentally incapable and treated accordingly, when they could make some decisions themselves. Or, if they are seen in a lucid period, they may be deemed competent and be left without enough support for significant decisions later. The British Medical Association and English Law Society have published a book on assessment of mental capacity[4] which provides more guidance.

Case example on assessing 'best interests'

C became progressively confused and was tearful and distressed when her doctor attempted to examine her. C had recurrent bowel problems and she was diagnosed as having bowel cancer, with local spread. A treatment decision had to be made in her best interests, as she was unable to express her own view. The health team could assess the clinical data but also needed to know something about her values and former wishes to decide how aggressively her cancer should be treated. Her family was asked what C would have wanted. As she had been a very religious woman, some relatives said that she would have seen the cancer as a facet of god's will, not to be resisted but others disagreed. This kind of topic had never been discussed. The possibility of surgery was explored but both the family and the health team were reluctant to expose her to painful treatment, which was beyond her comprehension. After discussion, it was agreed that from an objective perspective, her best interests lay in keeping her as comfortable as possible, providing palliative care and not subjecting her to repeated examinations or aggressive treatment which she was likely to resist. Efforts had rightly been made to ascertain her past wishes but these could not be sufficiently interpreted to cover a scenario she had never envisaged.

The law on proxy decision-making powers

Before the recent legislation in Scotland, England and Wales, there was no legal way anyone could give consent on behalf of an adult with impaired mental capacity. This is still the situation in Northern Ireland. The rest of the United Kingdom used to follow the common law system which Northern Ireland retains. Under this, treatment could go ahead where there was a 'necessity to act', and the action was in the patient's best interests. One of the major innovations of the legislation was to introduce proxy decision-making powers, enabling other people to make decisions on behalf of incapacitated adults. Any decision taken by a proxy must be based on an assessment either of best interests or benefit as laid out in the respective Acts. The legislation on proxy decision-making powers only applies to decisions on behalf of people who have lost capacity. While individuals retain mental capacity to make the decision in question, proxies cannot legally decide for them. For people facing incapacity, nominating a friend or relative to act as a proxy in future can be comforting but they need to consider carefully the nature and scope of the powers they are transferring. There is no obligation for anyone to nominate a proxy and if patients choose not to nominate someone, health professionals will carry out their own assessment of the individual's best interests. It is likely that proxy decision-makers will play an increasingly significant part in relation to the care and treatment of elderly incapacitated patients. Health professionals need to be aware of the duties and responsibilities of proxies. (See below and 'Further resources' listed at the end of the chapter.)

Proxy consent and refusal of treatment in England and Wales

Lasting powers of attorney

Before the Mental Capacity Act came into force in England and Wales, people could appoint someone to have power of attorney to manage their money or property if they themselves became mentally incapacitated, but not make their health decisions. The Act extended lasting powers of attorney (LPA) to cover health and welfare decisions. This includes authorising or refusing medical treatment on behalf of an incapacitated person. These powers of attorney also allow the nominated person to make personal welfare decisions for the incapacitated person, such as where the individual should live, aspects of daily care, social activities, personal correspondence and arrangements for community care services. People appointed as attorneys can play a considerable role in ensuring the welfare of older people who lack mental capacity.

Appointing an attorney

Competent adults can nominate another person – an attorney – to have an LPA and make health care decisions on their behalf when they themselves lose capacity. If they do so, they are known as 'donors' since they give decision-making power to someone. To be valid, the LPA must be a written document on a statutory form and must describe the nature and effect of the LPA. The document must be signed by the donor and the attorney. It must include a statement by an independent witness saying that the donor understands the LPA's purpose and makes it voluntarily. Decisions made by the attorney are then as valid as if made by the donor when competent. Donors have to specify if they want the attorney to be empowered to make health care decisions but, even if they do, the attorney cannot refuse life-sustaining treatment on the donor's behalf unless this is also explicitly stated in the LPA. Donors can choose one person to make all their decisions, or appoint several people to make different kinds of decisions or ask several people to act together. Donors can set conditions on the powers and can nominate replacement attorneys in case one dies or becomes unable to carry out the functions. An LPA cannot be used until it is registered with the Office of the Public Guardian. Donors can register the LPA while still mentally capable or the attorney can register it after the donor loses capacity.

A welfare LPA only comes into force when the donor loses capacity but problems can arise if it has not been registered by the time it is needed. It can take several weeks to register an LPA. If presented with an unregistered welfare LPA by relatives, doctors may have to apply to the Court of Protection for a court order if there is any disagreement about the proposed course of treatment (Ref. [2], Chapter 15).

Duties of attorneys

The Mental Capacity Act Code of Practice[2] provides detailed advice on LPAs and people acting as attorneys need to be familiar with it. They must make decisions in the best interests of the incapacitated person, which includes considering the donor's known wishes. They must also respect any restrictions or conditions imposed by the donor. Where possible, donors should be assisted to make the decision for themselves. In such cases, doctors may need to assess whether the donor has the mental capacity to make a particular decision (Ref. [2], Chapter 4). If the donor can make the health or welfare decision, a personal welfare LPA cannot be used. This is different from the situation for a property and affairs LPA, which can be used if the donor still has capacity, unless the donor specified otherwise. Before taking action under the LPA, attorneys must ensure that the LPA has been registered with the Public Guardian, as an unregistered LPA does not confer any powers.

Case example – arranging an LPA

B was worried that increasing forgetfulness was symptomatic of progressive mental decline. Controlling aspects of her life had always been important to her and she was distressed to think that matters were slipping out of her control. She appointed her eldest daughter as her welfare attorney to make future decisions if she became unable to decide for herself. She specified that her daughter should choose where B would live, the treatment she would receive and be able to refuse life-prolonging treatment if there were no likelihood of B regaining mental capacity. To ensure that her own views were implemented as much as possible, B not only discussed with her daughter how she wanted to be treated but also wrote copious notes covering every eventuality she could imagine. In fact, B retained her mental ability until she died and the LPA that she had carefully drawn up was never used. B's daughter said that the mental effort required to keep track of all the possible options had probably been a useful mental exercise for B over the years and helped keep her mind sharp. Although never needed for decision-making, the LPA had also given B a comforting sense of controlling the unpredictable end of life.

Role of health professionals regarding attorneys

When health professionals prepare care plans for patients who have appointed personal welfare attorneys, they must first assess whether the patients themselves can make the decision in question. If patients can decide the issue in question, their view prevails even though they may be confused on other matters. If patients lack capacity to make specific decisions, agreement for care or treatment must be sought from the attorney. Assessing what is in the patient's best interests also requires discussion with the attorney. The LPA allows attorneys to make decisions about medical treatment once the patient lacks capacity unless the LPA specifies otherwise. An attorney cannot consent to treatment if the patient made an advance refusal of it (a 'living will'), unless the LPA was made after the advance decision and clearly intended to transfer that decision to the attorney. If patients want their attorney to be able to refuse life-prolonging treatment, the LPA must specifically state that. If the health team do not believe that a decision about medical treatment taken by an attorney is in the best interests of the incapacitated individual, the case can be referred for adjudication to the Court of Protection.

Independent mental capacity advocates

In England and Wales, an independent advocacy scheme for particularly vulnerable incapacitated adults who lack other forms of support was implemented under the Mental Capacity Act. Where a decision is needed about serious medical treatment or place of residence for an incapacitated adult without friends, relatives, attorneys or a court-appointed deputy, an independent mental capacity advocate (IMCA) must be involved. IMCAs have legal obligations to take account of the Mental Capacity Act Code of Practice when making a decision on behalf of someone who is incapacitated. 'Serious medical treatment' includes providing, withdrawing or withholding treatment in circumstances where:

• there is a fine balance between the treatment's benefits, burdens and risks for the patient;
• there is a choice of treatments and it is unclear what would be best for the patient;
• what is proposed would involve serious consequences for the patient.

Practice for appointing IMCAs may vary from area to area but staff working in local authorities or the NHS must be able to identify when a patient needs an IMCA and know how to discuss the options with the IMCA. The first step is to know which organisation has been commissioned to provide an IMCA service in the area where the patient is currently living. Local authorities, Patient Advice and Liaison Service or a Citizens' Advice Bureau should hold such information. In Wales, Community Health Councils can provide it. The Department of Health's website has details of IMCA providers. Local arrangements govern how each IMCA service provider accepts referrals. Initially, this may be by phone or email. Criteria for referral are that:

- a person lacks the capacity to make the particular decision;
- the decision concerns serious medical treatment, a change in accommodation, a care review or an adult protection case;
- there is nobody who can appropriately support and represent the person (this does not apply to adult protection)[5].

Disputes, Court of Protection and Court-appointed deputies

The Mental Capacity Act created a new Court of Protection, which is the final arbiter about the legality of decisions made under the Act. The Court adjudicates if disagreements arise about what is in the best interests of an incapacitated adult. As well as deciding individual cases, the Court appoints deputies to assist with continued decision-making (Ref. [2], Chapter 8). An appointment order sets out the specific powers and scope of the deputy's authority. There are some general limitations: the most important being that deputies cannot make any decisions that the person concerned could make him- or herself. Where the individual clearly cannot make the decision personally, deputies must ensure their decisions are based upon the incapacitated individual's best interests. Deputies cannot refuse life-sustaining treatment on the individual's behalf. Nor can they go against a decision made by an attorney acting under an LPA, granted by the individual before losing capacity.

Case example – invoking the Court of Protection

F had appointed her husband as her attorney to make welfare decisions on her behalf. She was subsequently diagnosed with dementia and experienced quite rapid mental decline. Her husband continued to look after her at home, with help from social services. F's GP became concerned, however, when neighbours told him that the husband was not coping and had banned visitors, including the community services staff, from the house. The husband had said that F could not recognise them and the presence of strangers upset her. Neighbours reported disturbing noises and were worried that the husband might be hurting F. The GP arranged to visit and, despite an initially hostile reception, was able to talk to F's husband who was himself becoming confused and paranoid. The case was taken to the Court of Protection which requested a mental assessment of the husband. Although F had not been harmed, the court concluded that it was not in her best interests to be left in the care of her husband. Arrangements were made to transfer her to a care home, registered for the provision of dementia care. A deputy was appointed for her future care. Her husband remained at home and despite some confusion was considered competent, with some professional support, to manage his own life.

Proxy consent and refusal of treatment in Scotland

The Adults with Incapacity (Scotland) Act gives health professionals the authority to do what is reasonable and necessary to safeguard the health of an incapacitated adult. Detailed guidance on the Act is provided in the second edition of the Act's Code of Practice[3]. When competent, adults can appoint welfare attorneys with the power to make decisions on their behalf should they lose capacity later. Where a welfare attorney has been appointed, health professionals must seek that person's consent to treatment, except in emergencies. The Office of the Public Guardian (Scotland) holds a register of valid welfare attorneys.

General authority to treat

If an incapacitated adult has not nominated a proxy, doctors can issue a certificate of incapacity and make some decisions themselves under the Act's 'general authority to treat'. The certificate gives decision-making powers about treatment to the doctor who has signed it and to members of the health team. The certificate must specify how long it remains valid which can be up to 3 years for patients with severe dementia or profound learning disability. It is good practice for patients to be regularly reviewed. When issuing the certificate, doctors must have some treatment in mind, but it is not necessary to issue separate certificates for every intervention if the patient has multiple needs and the certificate can refer to an existing treatment plan. The general authority cannot be used where there is already a welfare attorney and it is reasonable for that person's views to be obtained. Similarly, if there is an appeal to the Court of Session regarding treatment, then only emergency treatment can be given until the Court has ruled.

Welfare attorneys and welfare guardians

In order to nominate a welfare attorney to make their future health decisions, competent adults need to understand what is involved and be free from undue influence. Alternatively, the Sheriff's court can either make an intervention order or appoint a welfare guardian with similar powers. Once an attorney or a guardian has been appointed, that person must be consulted about any proposed medical treatment where it is practical and reasonable to do so. Attorneys can consent to treatment on the patient's behalf as long as the proposed treatment fits the general principles set out earlier in this chapter.

Listening to relatives

For the care of incapacitated older people, it is usually important to involve individuals close to them. While duties of confidentiality and respect for patient privacy should be taken into account, it is generally accepted that relatives have a strong interest in the care of people who cannot speak for themselves. Finding out about the incapacitated person's wishes can sometimes be done by discussion with those close to the patient. The Adults with Incapacity (Scotland) Act also obliges health professionals to take account of the views of the patient's nearest relative and primary carer.

Disputes, the Sheriff and the Mental Welfare Commission

Although most decisions relating to incapacitated adults are not contested, situations arise in which genuine differences of opinion exist about whether a proposed treatment would be to the patient's benefit. Care providers may believe that relatives are not acting for the person's benefit, or relatives may think health professionals are not offering appropriate treatment choices. The Scottish legislation contains procedures for the resolution of disputes and these are explained in detail in the Code of Practice[3]. This sets out practical steps such as ensuring that relatives and carers are consulted and that such discussions are carefully documented in order to reduce the risk of long and costly court battles later. If, for example, health professionals propose a course of treatment for the incapacitated person which the welfare attorney refuses, the treatment cannot proceed until an opinion is obtained from a doctor appointed by the Mental Welfare Commission for Scotland. If the appointed doctor agrees that treatment should be given, it can proceed even if the attorney refuses. Any of the parties – including the attorney or other people with an interest in the patient's welfare – can apply to the Court of Session for a decision. If the welfare attorney asks on the patient's behalf for treatment which doctors consider inappropriate, an application can be made to the Sheriff to declare whether or not the treatment would benefit the patient.

Case example – resolving treatment disputes

W lived alone, with a large extended family nearby. After a fall, he was admitted to hospital where the health team diagnosed fluctuating mental capacity and early stage dementia. It was recommended that W should not be discharged home but that a place be found for him in a care home specialising in the care of dementia patients. This meant living at a distance from W's family. W was confused about the options. Good practice and the law required the health team to discuss them with W's relatives who felt strongly that W should remain in his own home. They said they would provide supervision for him as his dementia progressed and he should remain independent as long as possible, even though he might fall again. A dispute arose between the relatives and health team. If it could not be resolved through discussion, a decision would have to be sought from the Sheriff or the court. In the meantime, W experienced a period of lucidity in which he made it plain that he was determined to stay in his own home and accept the risks. His relatives drew up a rota of visitors and arranged for neighbours to keep an eye on W. Although the health team estimated that he would be safer and probably live longer in a residential home, W's own views were clearly against that and any future assessment of what would benefit him, as his capacity diminished, would need to take account of that.

Conscientious objection

In its discussion of dispute resolution, the Scottish Code of Practice makes clear that 'courts will not be able to instruct a practitioner to give a certain type of treatment against his or her principles – merely to instruct that the patient should receive that form of treatment' (Ref. [3], para 3.13).

Consent to treatment in Northern Ireland

There is no specific legislation relating to decision-making for incompetent adults in Northern Ireland. The legal position there is as it used to be in England and Wales before the Mental Capacity Act. It is governed by common law which says that nobody can consent to or refuse medical treatment on behalf of an adult who lacks mental capacity. Sometimes this is not fully understood by health professionals who spend time trying to find a relative to sign a consent form on behalf on an incapacitated adult. The fact that a relative's consent has no legal status is not always clear in hospital protocols. Treatment can be provided to an incapacitated adult without anyone's consent, if it is considered by the clinician in charge of the patient's care to be necessary and in the patient's best interests. The legal authority for this stems from a 1989 English case[6] in which the court clarified that necessary treatment can proceed where it would be in the best interests of an incapacitated adult, even though the patient cannot consent to it.

Participation in medical research

Competent patients can consent to participate in research, as long as they understand the implications, as is discussed at the start of this chapter. Although under-represented, older patients, including those with impaired capacity, can benefit in various ways from being involved in research. Frequent health checks and consistent attention can be beneficial and extra efforts can be made to eliminate minor problems that could interfere with the research data. A balance has to be struck between enabling research that benefits this population, while protecting the interests of a potentially vulnerable group.

Proxy consent to research in England and Wales

In the past, adults who were unable to give valid consent themselves could not participate unless the research would clearly be in their own best interests. In England and Wales, the Mental Capacity Act now permits the participation of incapacitated adults in some forms of medical research, including that which is deemed 'intrusive'. That is to say, it covers research that would be unlawful if it involved a mentally competent adult who had not given consent. (Clinical trials of new drugs are covered by separate rules, discussed later.) Researchers must ascertain whether the patient – although mentally impaired – can give a valid consent or refusal to being involved. If not, the general principles of the Act must be followed in terms of seeking the views of people close to the patient. The Mental Capacity Act Code of Practice (Ref. [2], Chapter 11) provides guidance on the sort of people who need to be consulted. It could be a relative or a person involved in the patient's care, provided it is not in a paid or professional capacity. A deputy appointed by the Court of Protection or an attorney acting under a registered LPA can be consulted about the patient's participation in research (unless they are acting in a paid or professional capacity). In addition, research involving incapacitated adults can only proceed if:

- it has research ethics committee approval;
- the research could not be carried out on competent adults;
- it is linked to the diagnosis or treatment of the condition from which the patient suffers;
- it considers the individual's interests;

- it is not contrary to the patient's interests and is likely either to benefit the patient or provide information to help others with similar conditions;
- risks are negligible and the benefits are in proportion to any burdens;
- any objections made by the incapacitated person must be respected.

Regulations have also been drawn up under the Act to cater for the management and protection of an adult enrolled in a research project who loses capacity after the research has commenced[7].

Proxy consent to research in Scotland
The Adults with Incapacity (Scotland) Act permits the involvement of incapacitated adults in research where the purpose is to gain knowledge about the causes, diagnosis, treatment or care of the patient's incapacity. The Act's Code of Practice provides details about the legal authority for research involving incapacitated adults (Ref. [3], section 4). The research should further knowledge and either directly benefit the patient or benefit other people with the same condition. In order for incapacitated adults to participate, the following conditions must also be met:
- consent from a proxy or the nearest relative is needed;
- the adult must show no objection;
- the research has ethics committee approval;
- it involves no or only minimal risk for the patient;
- it involves no or only minimal discomfort.

Research on incapacitated adults in Northern Ireland
In Northern Ireland, there is no statute covering this type of research and so participation of incapacitated adults is only clearly lawful if it is deemed to be in the best interests of the individual.

Medicines for human use (clinical trials) regulations

Participation in drug trials is regulated across the whole of the United Kingdom under the Medicines for Human Use (Clinical Trials) Regulations 2004 which permits the enrolment of mentally incapacitated adults in clinical trials relating to pharmaceutical products. As with any other research project, proposals must be approved by a research ethics committee. It must be impossible to do the research with competent, consenting adults. Before an incapacitated individual can be enrolled, somebody close to the patient who is willing to be consulted must agree to it. This could be a close relative or a welfare attorney. If neither exist, a proxy decision-maker who is independent of the research can authorise the participation of the incompetent adult. Additional safeguards are in place once the research is underway. If incapacitated individuals show distress or resistance or indicate by any means that they do not want to take part in the research, they must be withdrawn.

Case example on research

P's family were anxious that he be enrolled in research comparing different drugs to tackle the effects of dementia. P was unable to give valid consent but his son provided proxy authorisation. The family felt that participation was in P's best interests as it might give him early access to new medication. Even if he were randomly allocated to a placebo, they thought that regular chats with the research team and monitoring of his health could be beneficial. They hoped that if one of the drugs in the trial was successful, trial partici-pants would get preferential access. After a few weeks, however, P's behaviour changed. He became truculent and resisted efforts to take his blood pressure. The research team felt that he was objecting to the project and should be withdrawn. The family disagreed, as he seemed more lively and alert in the trial and not only would he lose the benefits of participation but would be ineligible to get early access to new drugs after the trial ended. The researcher and P's GP felt it would be illegal to allow P to continue as he was effectively displaying an objection. The family were told that, even if P continued in the trial until the end, he would not necessarily get any priority in getting the new drugs. That would be decided by factors, such as whether other patients with the condition were more needy or could benefit more from the drugs.

Human rights legislation

As we consider legislation that may be particularly relevant for the care of older people, we need to include the Human Rights Act 1998. It incorp-orates into UK law the rights set out in the European Convention on Human Rights and requires all 'public authorities', including professionals working for the NHS or Local Authorities, to act in accordance with those rights. Among the most relevant provisions for health and social care are:
• Article 2 – the right to life (which does not mean life must be prolonged at all costs)
• Article 3 – prohibition on inhuman or degrading treatment
• Article 5 – the right to liberty and security
• Article 8 – respect for private and family life, home and correspondence
• Article 14 – prohibition against discrimination.

In practice, there are various ways in which human rights legislation can particularly affect older people. The right to respect for private and family life is likely to be engaged in the placement of older people in residential care. A local authority, for example, who refuses to place married couples in the same nursing home, or who places individuals far from their family, could potentially breach their Article 8 right to respect for family life. If public authorities place restrictions on an individual's family life, they need to be able to justify their decision by showing that it is lawful, necessary and proportionate. The Act could be engaged in cases when treatment is withheld from a seriously ill patient or is given to a patient who has refused it. It could be engaged in situations where patients are refused treatment which could benefit them on the grounds of their age or their physical or mental disability. Other examples of how the care of older people could be affected by the human rights legislation are discussed in Chapters 6 and 7. Measures to detain or protect confused older people could amount to unlawful 'deprivation of liberty', contrary to Article 5 (see 'Bournewood case' in Chapter 6). Failure to take reasonable steps to provide artificial feeding at the end of life for a patient who is known to want it can also be argued under the human rights legislation (see 'Burke case' in Chapter 7). Although they are not the main theme of this report, issues such as 'undue delay' in providing treatment can also constitute a breach of human rights and can be argued in court under the human rights legislation, as is shown by the case of Mrs Watts, below.

Example of a legal case involving human rights

In October 2003, the High Court confirmed that where treatment cannot be provided without 'undue delay' in the United Kingdom, patients have the right to seek treatment in another EU member state and receive reimbursement of the cost from the NHS. Mrs Yvonne Watts was 72 years old and had osteoarthritis in both hips. She was originally told she would have to wait a year for the treatment she needed. She asked about receiving treatment in another country under the established procedures but was told that this was not possible because her waiting time was within the government's target and did not count as 'undue delay'. Mrs Watts arranged her operation privately in France and claimed reimbursement from the NHS. She argued that her human rights were relevant to the case in terms of Articles 3 and 8.

The court concluded that the authorities' refusal to fund treatment did not infringe her Article 3 or 8 rights. The 'ill-treatment' in question was not severe enough to engage her Article 3 rights. However, the court confirmed that 'undue delay' does not mean the same as being outside the government's waiting list targets and, although relevant, waiting lists are not determinative. In assessing what amounts to 'undue delay', all the circumstances of the individual case, including the patient's medical condition and, where appropriate, the degree of pain and the nature and extent of the person's disabilities, must be taken into consideration.

Yvonne Watts v (1) Bedford Primary Care Trust
(2) Secretary of State for Health[8]

In March 2008, the government pledged to extend the Human Rights Act to cover publicly funded residents in privately run residential and nursing homes. The Act puts on a legal footing what was already considered to be general good practice. It applies to everyone, regardless of age, disability, ethnicity or sexual orientation. In its most fundamental form, it involves seeing people as individuals whose rights and dignity demand respect. It is essential that decisions taken, both about individual patients and in terms of medical and social policy, take account of the Act. Although the fundamental concept of respecting people as individuals with moral and legal rights is straightforward, the application of human rights law is complex and often requires some interpretation. Its relevance to specific cases may not be immediately obvious. A good starting point from which to see the relevance of human rights to the care of older people is the report of the Joint Committee on Human Rights[9]. Among its main messages were statements about the need to respect dignity, avoid discrimination and promote equality. The report emphasised that the way in which older patients and care home residents are treated is not just a health or care issue but also a human rights issue. It criticised the 'embedded ageism within health care for older people' and said that 'there should be a positive duty on providers of health and residential care to promote equality for older people' (Ref. [9], pp. 24–5).

The British Medical Association has published general guidance[10] explaining how the law affects various aspects of medical practice and listing the types of cases that have so far been brought. It points out, for example, that withdrawing life-prolonging treatment, such as artificial nutrition and hydration, does not breach Article 2 – the right to life – if it is judged to be in the best interests of that individual. (This is discussed further in Chapter 8.)

Mental health legislation

As this chapter deals with consent and refusal in patient care, we need to mention, at least briefly, the main area of UK law where consent and refusal are not the key issues. Patients of any age who have a mental illness can be given treatment under compulsory mental health legislation. Unlike the mental capacity legislation which often affects older adults, the mental health legislation does not have a particular resonance for this patient population. While the mental health needs of older individuals must be taken into account and met, they are not generally significantly different in law to those of other patient groups with the same health problems.

It is not our intention, therefore, to provide a detailed commentary on the mental health law here, not least because three separate pieces of UK legislation deal with it and much of the law in this area is undergoing review. In England and Wales, the relevant legislation is the Mental Health Act 1983 as amended by the Mental Health Act 2007. In Scotland, it is the Mental Health (Care and Treatment) (Scotland Act) 2003. The Mental Health (Northern Ireland) Order 1986 is also currently undergoing review. These regulations provide a complex framework for the management of mentally disordered individuals and, in certain circumstances, they permit treatment to be given compulsorily despite a competent patient's refusal.

Summary of chapter

- *The law assumes that adults of any age can decide for themselves whether to accept or refuse care and treatment, unless there is evidence to the contrary.*
- *If older people have impaired or fluctuating mental capacity, they should still be involved as much as possible in decisions affecting them. They should be consulted when they are likely to be most lucid.*
- *If people have lost their mental capacity, the law (except in Northern Ireland) makes provision for various forms of proxy decision-making. Any decision made on behalf of a person lacking capacity must be based on their best interests (England, Wales and Northern Ireland) or what would benefit them (Scotland).*
- *Proxy consent applies to research as well as treatment decisions (except in Northern Ireland).*
- *The Human Rights Act is relevant for the day-to-day care of older people but is complex to interpret and expert legal advice is needed in some cases.*
- *There is sometimes a choice for health professionals to provide treatment under either the mental capacity legislative framework or the mental health framework. Both have some advantages and some drawbacks. In some circumstances, the law dictates which should be used.*

References

1. Some bodies, such as the Royal Colleges and the General Medical Council, recommend that written consent is obtained for certain types of procedure. Doctors should familiarise themselves with guidance relevant to their area of practice. The Department of Health publishes a series of model consent forms.
2. Department for Constitutional Affairs (2007). *Mental Capacity Act 2005 Code of Practice.* The Stationery Office Ltd, London.
3. Healthcare Policy & Strategy Directorate (2008). *Adults with Incapacity (Scotland) Act 2000, Code of Practice: Second Edition. For Practitioners Authorised to Carry Out Medical Treatment and Research Under Part 5 of the Act.* The Scottish Government, Edinburgh.
4. British Medical Association and The Law Society (2004). *Assessment of Mental Capacity: Guidance for Doctors and Lawyers: Second Edition.* BMJ Books, London. Third edition due 2009.
5. This is taken from: Office of the Public Guardian (2007). OPG06 *Making Decisions. The Independent Mental Capacity Advocate (IMCA) Service.* OPG, London, p. 25.
6. Re F (mental patient sterilisation) sub nom F v W Berkshire HA [1989] 2 All ER 545.
7. The Mental Capacity Act 2005 (Loss of Capacity During Research Project) (England) Regulations 2007. Mental Capacity Act 2005 (Loss of Capacity During Research Project) (Wales) Regulations 2007.
8. R (on the application of Yvonne Watts) v (1) Bedford Primary Care Trust (2) Secretary of State for Health. [2003] EWHC 2228.
9. House of Lords, House of Commons, Joint Committee on Human Rights (2007). *The Human Rights of Older People in Healthcare, Eighteenth Report of Session 2006–07. Volume 1 – Report and Formal Minutes.* The Stationery Office Ltd, London.
10. British Medical Association (2007). *The Impact of the Human Rights Act 1998 on Medical Decision-Making.* BMA, London.

Further resources

British Medical Association (2007). *The Impact of the Human Rights Act 1998 on Medical Decision-Making.* BMA, London.
British Medical Association (2008). *Mental Capacity Act Tool Kit.* BMA, London.
Department for Constitutional Affairs (2007). *Mental Capacity Act 2005 Code of Practice.* The Stationery Office Ltd, London.
Healthcare Policy & Strategy Directorate (2008). *Adults with Incapacity (Scotland) Act 2000, Code of Practice: Second Edition. For Practitioners Authorised to Carry Out Medical Treatment and Research Under Part 5 of the Act.* The Scottish Government, Edinburgh.

Chapter 5 **Privacy and confidentiality**

Older people's right to privacy

In health care, the professional duty of confidentiality is usually associated with protection of sensitive health care information. In communal environments, confidentiality can be hard to protect. Individuals and their families may not have the space to talk in private, and sensitive medical advice is sometimes delivered where other people can overhear[1]. Important as confidentiality is, it is not the only aspect of people's rights to privacy in healthcare settings and residential facilities. These rights are more wide-ranging. Professionals providing care for older people, especially for individuals experiencing mental confusion, need to be aware of ways in which the dignity and privacy of those individuals can be inadvertently undermined. The importance of privacy is well recognised in law. Article 8 of the Human Rights Act 1998 (the HRA) provides for 'the right to respect for (an individual's) private and family life'.

In hospital settings, mixed-sex wards and mixed accommodation involve a lack of privacy which the Parliamentary Human Rights Committee considered could constitute a breach of Article 8 of the HRA[1]. It is difficult to ensure privacy and dignity in mixed wards, particularly when patients are partially clothed or naked[2]. Shared bathing and toilet facilities also raise concern about lack of privacy, especially when patients are unable to use the toilet in private. This was a key message from the British Geriatrics Society (2006) Dignity Behind Closed Doors campaign.

Dignity is undermined by practices such as care home residents being fed whilst on a commode[1]. In England, National Minimum Standards for privacy and dignity in social care services were introduced in 2003. In 2006, the Commission for Social Care Inspection reported significant improvement by social care and residential services in meeting those standards[3]. Nevertheless, it still indicated that 21% of care homes were failing to do so. One of the findings from the Healthcare Commission's 2007 inspection report on acute hospital trusts was that the core standard relating to patient

The Ethics of Caring for Older People 2nd Edition. By British Medical Association. Published 2009 by Blackwell Publishing Limited, ISBN 9781405176279.

dignity was the standard most at risk of not being met. This was mainly due to lack of single-sex accommodation, including single-sex washing and toilet facilities[4]. All individuals are entitled to have their privacy respected in health and care settings. They should have access to private and dignified toilet facilities[5].

The professional and legal duty of confidentiality

Individuals are entitled to expect that their identifiable health information is kept confidential unless there is a compelling reason why it should not be. That does not mean it cannot be shared with people close to that person or with professionals providing care and support. Patients generally want essential information to be available to the team caring for them and this form of disclosure is usually governed by implied consent. People should be explicitly asked, however, whether they want information about their care, prognosis and treatment shared with their relatives or friends.

All identifiable health information health professionals acquire in a professional capacity is subject to the duty of confidentiality. There are three broad exceptions:

1. where the patient gives consent to others being informed;
2. where the law requires disclosure of the information;
3. where there is an overriding public interest.

In addition to the ethical duty of confidentiality, doctors receiving information in order to provide support and care for a patient are also bound by a legal duty of confidence. They also have obligations to ensure that patient information that they record is securely stored.

Legal sources of confidentiality rights and protections

The legal position on the confidentiality of health information is complex. Its use is governed by:

- *Data Protection Act 1998 (the DPA) – its purpose is to protect the right of individuals to privacy with respect to the processing of personal data. It is not always understood that the DPA 'permits' but does not 'require' the release of information. The Act requires organisations to process fairly and lawfully any information which might enable an individual to be identified. Individuals have a right to know what information about them is being processed and when (the 'fair processing' requirement) and they have rights of access to personal information stored about them. The processing itself must meet the legal standards, including the common law duty of confidentiality. This has a bearing on the need for patients to give consent before identifying health information is* shared. The DPA also requires organisations that wish to process identifying data to use the minimum of information necessary and to retain it only for as long as is needed for the purpose for which it was originally collected.

- HRA 1998 – a right to 'respect for private and family life' is guaranteed in Article 8 of the HRA. This right is not absolute, and may be derogated from where the law permits and 'where necessary in a democratic society in the interests of national security, public safety or the economic well-being of the country, for the prevention of disorder or crime, for the protection of health or morals or for the protection of the rights and freedoms of others'. The effect is similar to that of the common law: privacy is an important principle which must be respected but may be breached where other significant interests prevail. Any such breach must be both necessary and proportionate to the benefits/harms it is intended to bring/avoid.
- The Common Law – this is based on previous judgments in court. Whilst the common law may be interpreted in various ways, it is widely accepted that it reinforces the view that information may be disclosed with patient consent, where there is a public interest or where the law requires it.
- In England and Wales, Section 251 of the NHS Act 2006 gives the Secretary of State for Health power to make regulations permitting the disclosure of identifiable information without the individual's consent in some circumstances. This may be to support essential NHS activity or for medical purposes that are in the interests of the wider public, where obtaining consent is not feasible and anonymised information will not suffice. Health professionals can apply to the Patient Information Advisory Group, an independent public body which advises the Secretary of State on the lawful basis for disclosure of patient-identifiable information.
- NHS Care Record Guarantee – this sets out the rules governing electronically held information on the NHS Care Records Service. The guarantee covers patients' access to their own records, controls on access by others, how access is monitored and policed, patients' options to further limit access, access in an emergency and what happens when patients cannot make decisions for themselves.
- Professional Standards – all health professionals must maintain the standards of confidentiality laid down by their professional body, such as the General Medical Council (GMC) for doctors and the Nursing and Midwifery Council (NMC) for nurses.
- Policies and Organisational Standards – a wide range of these exist to advise health professionals and ensure that patients are made aware about the use of their information about them. (The main ones are listed under 'Further resources' at the end of this chapter.)

Consent to disclosure

Individuals' consent to disclosure of information can be limited to sharing specific information with a particular person or organisation for a defined purpose or general consent to future disclosure for various purposes. Such consent should be informed, voluntary and may need to be documented, depending on the gravity of the implications of disclosure and the sensitivity of the information. Consent to disclosure can be explicit or implied. Explicit (or express) consent occurs when a person actively agrees verbally or in writing to a defined use or disclosure of information. The advantage of explicit consent is that there is no doubt as to what has been agreed. Consent to disclosure can also be implied by a person's behaviour but in order to be valid, individuals must be aware what information about them will be shared, with whom and for what purpose. They must also know that they can refuse to disclose it. If they are relying on a patient's implied consent to justify disclosure, health professionals must be able to demonstrate why they believe the individual implicitly consented. If there is no good reason to believe that the person did, the disclosure is without consent and some other justification is needed to permit it. In addition to discussions about disclosure in the course of a doctor–patient consultation, leaflets, posters and information with hospital appointment letters can inform patients about information sharing and give them an opportunity to opt out. A combination of methods is more likely to ensure that patients are aware.

Refusal to allow disclosure

All competent patients can object to information they provide in confidence being disclosed, even if disclosure is to another professional providing care. In exceptional circumstances, some patients refuse to allow certain information to be divulged to other health professionals treating them. This means that they risk receiving substandard care because the health team caring for them lacks the full facts. If patients understand this and any other consequences of their choice, their wishes must be respected, unless disclosure is required by law or there is an overriding public interest in disclosure.

Case example – refusal of disclosure

A was a widower, living alone. His daughter lived abroad and had only sporadic contact with him. When she became concerned about A's health, the daughter asked A's GP about his medical condition, knowing that A regularly saw his GP. The GP talked to A about the daughter's request but A was unwilling to have his health information shared with her. Since A was mentally competent, the GP informed A's daughter that no information could be disclosed without her father's explicit consent.

Disclosure to other health professionals

In the absence of evidence to the contrary, patients are normally considered to have given implied consent for health professionals to share information within the health team for the purpose of their care. The criteria for implied consent, mentioned earlier, must be met and so patients must generally be aware that their information will be shared within the care team, unless they object. Even if patients do not object, health and care professionals should only share what is necessary and relevant for the individual's care, on a 'need-to-know' basis. Patients' refusal to allow information sharing with health professionals treating them may mean that they receive poorer quality care and risk their own safety, but an informed refusal by a competent person should be respected (unless disclosure is required by law or by the public interest). Competent individuals can risk their own health but not that of other people and so information about serious infectious conditions, for example, methicillin-resistant *Staphylococcus aureus*, can generally be shared if essential to protect others. Health and social care, although often closely related, may have different criteria and thresholds for the disclosure of confidential information. Disclosure of their health information to social services usually requires explicit consent from competent patients (see the next section).

Disclosure in multi-agency working

Various aspects of liaison between people providing care are touched upon in Chapter 2 where effective communication is emphasised. Here we consider the other side of the picture and focus on limiting information to respect patient confidentiality. A balance needs to be found which facilitates essential information sharing to benefit older people whilst recognising their rights to privacy. The care of older people is often shared between health professionals and agencies such as social services and housing and benefits agencies. Occasionally, other partners are also involved, such as multi-agency protection panels and the police. In community settings, many integrated teams include workers from health, social services and non-statutory bodies. These various agencies may have different approaches to the disclosure of confidential information and so it is important to have agreed policies on information sharing which encourage effective multi-agency working within defined and clearly understood boundaries. Health information is generally seen as special, sensitive and subject to more restrictions than some other personal information. Health professionals should talk to their patients about the desirability of sharing essential health information with other agencies, where appropriate. A range of service providers may need to be involved in discussions about older patients' needs in case conferences or multidisciplinary meetings. In such circumstances, competent patients should be aware of, and consent to, the sharing of any confidential personal health information. In the case of older people with impaired mental capacity, information should be shared when that would be in their best interests. If there is neither consent nor a best interests justification for information sharing, disclosure of identifiable personal health information should only occur when required by law or by the public interest. As is discussed later, evidence of abuse or neglect of older people is the kind of exceptional circumstance that may allow disclosure in the public interest, even if the individual is reluctant to allow it.

Disclosure to friends, relatives and next of kin

The same duty of confidentiality is owed to all patients, irrespective of age or disability. Competent older people can say whom they want kept informed about their health and welfare. It is for them to decide if and how they allow the sharing of their information. It is not unusual, however, for relatives to request that some diagnostic information is given to them alone, to avoid distressing the patient. As is discussed in Chapter 2, it is important to explain that the duty of the health care team is to the patient, who should be able to exercise his or her own preference. When older people lack mental capacity, it is usually reasonable to assume that they would want people close to them to be kept informed, unless there is evidence to the contrary. This does not, however, mean that all information should be routinely shared. If the information is particularly sensitive, a judgement is needed about how much the individual would have wanted passed on and to whom. If there is evidence that the person who is now incompetent did not want information shared, this must be respected. Those close to patients lacking capacity have an important part to play in decision-making, whether they have a formal role as a proxy decision-maker (see patients who lack capacity later) or more informally in terms of helping the health care team to assess the patient's best interests. They may be unable to carry out these roles without some information about the patient's medical condition.

Despite the widespread use of the phrase 'next of kin', the term is neither defined nor has legal status. The next of kin cannot give or withhold consent to the sharing of information on a patient's behalf. Nor do they have rights of access to medical records or information about a patient's medical condition. The next of kin cannot make decisions on behalf of a patient who lacks capacity. If, however, patients name somebody they trust as a next of kin (who may not necessarily be any relation) and give the health team the permission to discuss care options with that person, this can be helpful for staff looking after the patient. There are no rules about who can be considered next of kin, as long as the patient agrees that this is the person who should be consulted in case of need. It is important not to confuse the undefined concept of next of kin with the very specific role of the 'nearest relative' under the Mental Health Act, which is subject to the statutory provisions of the Act.

Disclosure to solicitors

Doctors and lawyers often need to liaise if it is suspected that an older person lacks sufficient mental capacity to make a specific decision. Doctors are often asked, for example, to certify whether patients have capacity to make or alter their will or donate their assets to relatives in their lifetime[6]. The law assumes they have, unless there is evidence to the contrary but, in cases of doubt, an assessment needs to be carried out. The results can be disclosed to the solicitor with the consent of a patient found to be competent or in the best interests of a patient with impaired capacity. Health records required for legal proceedings are usually obtained via an application under the DPA 1998. Health professionals releasing information to lawyers acting for their patients should ensure that they have the patient's written consent to disclosure and that the patient understands the nature and extent of the information disclosed. In practice, most solicitors provide a copy of the patient's signed consent when requesting confidential information. If a solicitor acting for another party seeks information about a patient, the patient's consent to the disclosure must be obtained. If the patient refuses, the solicitor may apply for a court order requiring disclosure of the information.

Disclosure for spiritual care

As is discussed in Chapter 8, spiritual care is provided by a range of counsellors and advisers. Some people are happy for information about their needs and affiliations to be passed to a chaplain, rabbi, imam or humanist adviser who may then arrange spiritual care. Information about affiliation and clinical information about an individual's health should not be passed on without that person's consent. If patients lack the capacity to give consent, those close to the patient should be consulted to explore the patient's wishes, feelings and beliefs prior to any disclosure of information.

Disclosure to pursue a complaint

When individuals initiate a complaint about health or social care, it is unlikely that an investigation can take place without access to relevant parts of their record. The use of some identifiable information is necessary and appropriate, but individuals should be made aware of who will see information about them and the safeguards in place to minimise risks to confidentiality. Guidance on maintaining confidentiality in the NHS complaints procedures is available from the health departments. Sometimes people involve their MP or other elected representative in the complaints process. Where the MP states in writing that the individual has consented to disclosure, this may usually be accepted without further reference to the patient. People may also authorise relatives or carers to act on their behalf in pursuance of a complaint. Health professionals who are asked to disclose information in these circumstances must be satisfied that the individual has consented to the disclosure.

Individuals who lack mental capacity to consent to disclosure

Adults are assumed to have the capacity to make their own decisions, unless evidence indicates the contrary. Many people living with a mental impairment or fluctuating capacity can make valid decisions about disclosure. If an individual lacks the mental capacity to decide about disclosure at the time the decision has to be made, an assessment is needed of what would be in that person's best interests or what would benefit the individual. (The legislation in Scotland talks about 'benefit', whereas the 'best interests' of the incapacitated person are the legal criteria in the rest of the United Kingdom; see Chapter 3.) The various types of disclosure mentioned earlier in relation to competent people may also arise for people with impaired competence, and the criteria justifying the disclosure are that it would benefit the individual or is in that person's best interests. When patients lack capacity, health professionals may need to share information with relatives, friends or carers to enable them to assess the patient's best interests in a particular situation.

Case example – disclosure in an individual's best interests

D was resident in a care home. The care home manager received a request from D's son to see D's medical records. The son was worried that the home was unable to meet D's needs since he was becoming confused. Aware of the duty of confidentiality to D, the manager asked for advice from D's doctor who judged that D was unable to understand the issues due to deteriorating mental abilities and could not consent to disclosure. The manager saw no reason why D would have objected to information being shared with his son and, given the fact that the son was so worried, it seemed it would be in D's 'best interests' to disclose his file. The doctor agreed that it was appropriate to give D's son the information necessary for him to act in D's best interests but felt that it was inappropriate to disclose the whole of D's medical records relating to his former life, as some of this was sensitive information. The doctor, therefore, advised the manager to allow D's son access to current and relevant information from the file but not the entire record.

Sharing information with proxy decision-makers

When patients lack mental capacity, health professionals are likely to need to share information with any individual authorised to make proxy decisions. Chapter 4 points out how in England and Wales the Mental Capacity Act provides for the appointment of welfare attorneys to make proxy health and welfare decisions. The Court of Protection can also appoint deputies to do so. The goal of the Act is to empower individuals and people acting on their behalf. This may entail giving access to relevant parts of the incapacitated person's medical record, unless health professionals can demonstrate that it would not be in the patient's best interests. If such a case arose where it seemed not to be in the patient's best interests, the Court of Protection could adjudicate as to whether the records should be released. When patients lack capacity and have no relatives or friends to be consulted, an Independent Mental Capacity Advocate should be appointed. An attorney or deputy can also be appointed to make decisions relating to the management of property and financial affairs. Disclosure of information about the patient to these decision-makers is based on an assessment of the patient's best interests. In Northern Ireland, there is no mental capacity legislation but the common law also operates on the basis of an assessment of the patient's best interests.

Chapter 4 covers in more detail the situation in Scotland, where the Adults with Incapacity (Scotland) Act allows for the appointment of welfare attorneys. The Court of Session can also appoint deputies to make health and welfare decisions. An attorney or deputy can also be appointed to make decisions relating to the management of property and financial affairs. In Scotland, the standard for assessing whether an action or a disclosure on behalf of an incapacitated adult is appropriate is based on whether it would 'benefit' that person. As Chapter 4 discusses, 'benefit' and 'best interests' are very similar concepts. In all of the cases mentioned earlier, health professionals can only disclose information about the incapacitated person to proxy decision-makers on the basis of the patient's best interests or to provide benefit. That does not mean that they always need access to the whole patient record but they need to have relevant information to deal with the issue in question.

Case example – disclosure to a welfare attorney

B had early stage dementia but managed at home, with support from social services. A fall, however, resulted in a broken hip and B was admitted to hospital. Her daughter had been appointed earlier as B's welfare attorney and she felt that B's overall health had deteriorated, requiring B to be cared for in a residential setting. A dispute arose between B's daughter and the discharge team about appropriate accommodation for B, who lacked capacity to make the decision herself. B's daughter asked to see her mother's health and social care records but initially this request was refused by the hospital on the grounds that it breached B's confidentiality. When it was pointed out that B's daughter was a welfare attorney and that she needed information to decide B's future care, the hospital sought legal advice. This confirmed that the relevant records should be promptly released to B's daughter. It might have been equally possible to release relevant information on 'best interests' grounds but the fact that legal steps had been taken to appoint a welfare attorney made the situation unambiguously clear.

Legal and statutory disclosures

Some disclosures are required by law, regardless of patient consent or whether the individual is mentally competent. Such statute and regulations deal primarily with disclosures to avert potential dangers to society from serious communicable diseases and disclosures in the interests of order and justice. Under public health legislation, for example, doctors must notify local authorities of the identity, sex and address of people with a notifiable disease, including food poisoning. Deaths, major injuries, certain accidents and diseases and dangerous occurrences must be reported under health and safety legislation. Health and care professionals must be aware of their obligations to disclose in these circumstances. Where a statutory requirement exists, consent is not necessary as individuals have no right to refuse but they should be aware that disclosure to a secure authority is required.

The courts, including the coroner's courts, some tribunals and bodies appointed to hold enquiries such as the GMC, have legal powers to require disclosure, without the individual's consent, of information relevant to matters within their jurisdiction. Applications for court orders must be served on the individual who must have an opportunity to make representations to the court, if he or she objects to the disclosure of their information. Health professionals are justified in disclosing information in response to a court order when they believe that they have information falling within the category specified by the order. Failure to comply with a court order to release records may be an offence, but health professionals should object to the judge or presiding officer if they believe that the records contain information that should not be disclosed. This may be the case, for example, if the record has information about third parties unconnected with the proceedings.

Disclosure in the public interest

In some cases, identifiable information can be shared with third parties if disclosure is justifiable in the 'public interest'. The right to confidentiality is never absolute and may be overridden when the rights of others are jeopardised in a serious way. When the rights of different parties collide, a balance must be stuck between respecting confidentiality and averting harm by breaching it. Disclosures in the public interest are based on the common law and occur when disclosure is essential to prevent a serious threat to public health or to national security, or a risk of serious harm to someone or to prevent or detect a serious crime. The regulatory body for medicine, the GMC, states:

> *Disclosure of personal information without consent may be justified in the public interest where failure to do so may expose the patient or others to risk of death or serious harm. Where the patient or others are exposed to a risk so serious that it outweighs the patient's privacy interest, you should seek consent to disclosure where practicable. If it is not practicable to seek consent, you should disclose information promptly to an appropriate person or authority. You should generally inform the patient before disclosing the information. If you seek consent and the patient withholds it you should consider the reasons for this, if any are provided by the patient. If you remain of the view that disclosure is necessary to protect a third party from death or serious harm, you should disclose information promptly to an appropriate person or authority*[7].

Similarly, the Nursing and Midwifery Council's code of professional conduct states that nurses should protect all confidential information and make disclosures without consent only where required by law or order of a court or where disclosure can be justified in the wider public interest[8].

> **Case example – disclosure in the public interest**
>
> In his late sixties, P suffered from a serious heart condition and experienced occasional bouts of dizziness, fainting and blackouts. He lived in a rural area and the use of a car to see friends, family and do his weekly shopping contributed greatly to his quality of life. Although P had never passed out while driving, this was a possibility which posed a risk of serious harm to himself and others. P's GP understood how important driving was for P but she urged him to stop. He promised to reduce the use of his car, only driving occasionally but the doctor made clear that if P did not voluntarily stop, she would have to talk to the Driving and Vehicle Licensing Authority (DVLA) about him. This eventually persuaded P to stop driving and disclose his heart condition to the DVLA. P's GP put him in touch with a voluntary organisation which could arrange transport for him. Through frank discussion with his GP, P voluntarily gave up driving. Had he not, P's GP would have had to consider breaching confidentiality and disclosing his heart condition to the DVLA. Such disclosure to the DVLA by health professionals is not mandatory, but non-disclosure could leave them open to a charge of negligence if harm resulted and it was known that the patient himself or herself would not take action.

Decisions to disclose in the public interest are based on a balancing of several moral imperatives, including the duty to minimise the risk of harm occurring if no disclosure is made and the duty to avoid, if possible, the harms associated with breaching the patient's confidentiality. Wherever possible, the patient should be urged to take responsibility for making the disclosure voluntarily. Breaching confidentiality without consent has implications for the doctor–patient relationship and for public trust in a confidential health service but is sometimes unavoidable. Decisions to disclose health information in the 'public interest' should be taken by the clinician with overall responsibility for the patient's care and should involve the minimum of information necessary to deal with the risk. Careful thought must be given to the question of who should be given the information, and health professionals must be prepared to justify their decision to the GMC or other disciplinary body.

Disclosure of information in relation to suspected abuse of older people

A difficult aspect of disclosure in the public interest can arise in relation to disclosures about abuse. As is discussed in Chapter 2, neglect is the most common form of mistreatment of older people. This is sometimes unintentional, stemming from lack of awareness, insufficient training or poor communication among care providers about the older person's needs for assistance. Neglect in such situations needs to be reported and immediately addressed. Disclosure and investigation of poor standards, as steps towards instituting measures to improve care, are ethically straightforward in such situations. Specific disclosures about identifiable individuals should still be discussed with them but the need for proper investigation is usually accepted by all concerned. Awareness is also increasing of the fact that older people can be subjected to deliberate and secretive physical, psychological or financial abuse by relatives or carers. General issues of how to raise with patients the question of such suspected abuse are discussed in Chapter 2. Here we focus on situations where the individual's confidentiality may need to be breached. Where abuse or neglect is suspected, care professionals need to talk sensitively to the person concerned, document their concerns, talk to a line manager and take expert advice from someone like a local Safeguarding Adults Co-ordinator. (Further resources of expert advice on abuse of older people are given at the end of this chapter.) Depending on the evidence and the consensus of opinion, consideration may need to be given to the involvement of other agencies, including social services and the police.

Mentally competent individuals

Sensitive discussion about the possibility of abuse or neglect needs to take place with the individual suspected of having suffered it. This may lead to disclosures and, if so, it is vital to plan with the individual how these will be handled. It is important to ensure that individuals retain as much control as possible over disclosures of information about themselves while ensuring that nobody's safety is jeopardised by delays. People exposed to abuse may initially feel threatened or embarrassed about other people knowing or they may be worried that disclosure will lead to further maltreatment. If the perpetrator of abuse is a family member, older people may feel a misplaced sense of loyalty or worry about the effects of disclosure on other family members. They may need time to come to a firm decision about disclosure but it is obviously important that, in the interim, prompt steps are taken to protect their safety. This may mean postponing a discharge from hospital or arranging some intermediate care until other arrangements can be made. Some people who have endured threats or violence need counselling and repeated consultations. Care for older people is often provided by multidisciplinary teams and suspicions of abuse or neglect are likely to need liaison with other members of the team. Providing that competent patients consent, their situation can be discussed with other people. In some situations, advice can be sought from external expert sources without necessarily disclosing the individual's identity.

Competent individuals have the right to object to information they gave in confidence being disclosed in a form that identifies them. In most situations, if they do not wish to have their information shared with other carers or agencies, those wishes should be respected. Secrecy should not be promised, however, as there are limits to the right of confidentiality. Where evidence of abuse or neglect exists, inaction is not an option. Abuse or neglect in a nursing home or residential institution is likely to mean that other vulnerable people are at risk. In that case, disclosure in the public interest is likely to be required. In a family home, domestic violence involving older people may mean that others in the household are at risk. Decisions have to be made on a case-by-case basis, but abuse and neglect can amount to serious harm or a serious crime. In such exceptional circumstances, disclosure contrary to the individual's wishes may be justified in the public interest but is a last resort when counselling and encouragement fail. Disclosure must be to a reputable agency or statutory body and only relevant information should be provided. Where there is any doubt as to whether disclosure would be in the public interest, care providers should discuss the matter with a senior colleague, the Trust's legal team, an external expert, professional body or defence organisation. Health professionals must ensure that their concerns, including any discussions a with the patient, colleagues or professionals in other agencies are clearly recorded.

Patients with impaired mental competence

Where health professionals have concerns about a person lacking capacity, who is or may be at risk of abuse or neglect, it is essential that these concerns are acted upon promptly. Information should be given to an appropriate person or statutory body, in order to prevent further harm. In virtually all cases, it is likely to be in the individual's best interests that action is taken as promptly as possible but if there is any doubt as to whether disclosure is justifiable, advice should be sought from the same sources as mentioned earlier.

General management of confidential data

What information is confidential?

All information which identifies patients or clients of social services and gives details about them is confidential. This includes their name and address, medical records, photographs, videos, audiotapes and anything else that identifies them directly or indirectly. Records of rare diseases, for example, or drug treatments or statistical analyses which have very small numbers within a small population may allow individuals to be identified, even though they are not named. If identifiable information is needed for administrative, planning, teaching or research purposes by third parties, the patient's consent should be obtained. Anonymised information should be used wherever possible for such purposes (see 'Secondary uses of patient information' on page 73).

The duty to keep identifiable information secure

Confidential patient information needs to be protected against external threats such as theft and internal threats such as inappropriate access by unauthorised staff. Computers, medical records or files should not be left unattended. Ideally, all records and laptops containing patient data should be in a locked environment and not removed from the workplace. Where it is essential to move records, for example when doctors visit patients in nursing homes, safeguards must be in place. In nursing homes and other residential facilities, medical and other personal information must also be stored securely with clear rules about who has access. Discussion about the management of patients should be out of earshot of anyone not involved in their care. All employees who come into contact with personal health information should be trained in confidentiality and security issues and be aware of their ethical, legal and contractual duties of confidentiality.

Anonymisation and pseudonymisation

Information can be used more freely for purposes such as research, teaching or service planning if it does not identify individuals. Usually, information is considered to be anonymous if clinical or administrative details are separated from anything that might permit the individual to be identified such as name, date of birth and postcode. Even when such obvious identifiers are removed, rare diseases or drug treatments and statistical analyses which have very small numbers may allow people to be identified. A combination of details increases the chance of identification. Health professionals must anonymise information if releasing it without patient consent when there is no other overriding justification for disclosure. It is not necessary to seek consent for use of anonymised data but patients should generally be informed about it.

Pseudonymisation is often referred to as reversible anonymisation. Patient identifiers such as name, address or NHS number are substituted with a pseudonym, code or other unique reference so that the data are only identifiable to those who have the code. When people using the data have no means to reverse the process and identify individuals, the data can be treated as anonymised and there is no requirement to seek consent. Pseudonymised data are commonly used in research and patients should generally be informed about that.

Secondary uses of patient information

Health information is collected primarily to provide individuals' treatment and care but it also has ancillary or secondary purposes, such as service planning, commissioning and payment, audit, administration, research and education. No breach of confidentiality occurs if the secondary use is carried out by professionals who already have access to the information for the provision of care. For example, audit and planning can be undertaken within a health team. Patients do not need to consent but should generally be aware of this.

Often, requests for health information for secondary purposes come from NHS employees outside the health team or from agencies commissioned to carry out projects for the NHS. Although patients expect that their information will be kept private, most people also recognise that society benefits from useful research, the training of health professionals and having effective services. What is often unclear is the extent to which individual rights to privacy should give way to the needs of society as a whole but various measures, such as the data protection legislation, are in place to balance out those values. Consent is normally needed if identifiable patient data are required for secondary uses but anonymised data which do not breach confidentiality nor require consent should be used wherever possible. (The British Medical Association has detailed guidance about secondary uses of health data on its website.)

Secure retention and disposal of records

NHS records are subject to minimum retention periods which apply to both electronic and manual records. Private doctors are advised to retain their records for the same periods as NHS records are kept. Health records should be stored for a minimum of 8 years after the last episode of care or 8 years after the patient's death. The records of mentally disordered persons (within the meaning of the Mental Health Act 1983) should be kept for a minimum of 20 years after the last entry, or 8 years after the patient's death. When health records are destroyed, the method must be effective and not compromise confidentiality. Incineration, pulping and shredding are appropriate for manual records. Electronic data should be destroyed using appropriate data destruction software.

Summary of chapter

- Older people have the same confidentiality rights as other people and should be consulted about disclosures of their information, including to their friends and relatives.
- Implied consent is normally sufficient for sharing their health information within the health team.
- When patients refuse disclosure, their wishes should normally be respected, unless the law requires disclosure or there is an overriding public interest.
- Evidence of abuse or neglect may trigger disclosure in the public interest but should be discussed with the individual.
- Disclosures should be kept to the minimum necessary to achieve the purpose.
- Health professionals must always be prepared to justify their decisions about the use and disclosure of personal health information.

References

1. House of Lords, House of Commons Joint Committee on Human Rights (2007). *The Human Rights of Older People in Healthcare. Eighteenth Report of Session 2006–07. Volume 1 – Report and Formal Minutes.* The Stationery Office Ltd, London.
2. House of Lords, House of Commons Joint Committee on Human Rights (2007). *The Human Rights of Older People in Healthcare. Eighteenth Report of Session 2006–07. Volume 2 – Oral and Written Evidence.* The Stationery Office Ltd, London.
3. Commission for Social Care Inspection (2008). *State of Social Care Report 2005–06.* CSCI, London.
4. Healthcare Commission (2007). *Caring for Dignity: A National Report on Dignity in Care for Older People While in Hospital.* Commission for Healthcare Audit and Inspection, London.
5. The British Geriatrics Society (2006). *Dignity Behind Closed Doors Campaign.*
6. The third edition of the BMA and Law Society book *Assessment of Mental Capacity* sets out checklists for assessing capacity for various legal purposes.
7. General Medical Council (2004). *Confidentiality: Protecting and Providing Information.* GMC, London, para 27.
8. Nursing and Midwifery Council (2008). *The NMC Code of Professional Conduct: Standards for Conduct, Performance and Ethics.* NMC, London.

Further resources

Association of Directors of Adult Social Services (2005). *Safeguarding Adults: A National Framework of Standards for good practice and outcomes in adult protection work.* ADASS, London.

British Geriatric Society (2006). *Behind Closed Doors: Using the Toilet in Private.* BGS, London.

Department of Health and Home Office (2000). *No secrets: Guidance on developing and implementing multi-agency policies and procedures to protect vulnerable adults from abuse.* DH and HO, London.

Department of Health (2006). *The Caldicott Guardian Manual.* DH, London.

General Medical Council (2004). *Confidentiality: Protecting and Providing Information.* GMC, London.

NHS Institute for Innovation and Improvement (2008). *Privacy and Dignity: The Elimination of Mixed Sex Accommodation, a Good Practice Guide and Self.* NHS Institute for Innovation and Improvement, London.

The Health Departments for England, Wales, Scotland and Northern Ireland publish guidance on confidentiality. Contact details for each of the Departments are provided in 'Useful Organisations', at the end of this book.

The Information Commissioner (2002). *Guidance on the Use and Disclosure of Health Data. Guidance on the Application of the Data Protection Act.* ICO, London.

Chapter 6 Consent to use of protective measures and restraint

Balancing liberty and protection

The care of older patients with impaired mental capacity raises ethical and practical dilemmas. For this population, some protective measures are likely to be needed to keep them safe but such measures need to be proportionate to the risk and seriousness of the anticipated harm. Wherever possible, they need to be discussed with the individuals concerned, who should be given support to make their own decisions if they can. People with impaired capacity are not the only group for whom restrictions and safeguards are routinely used. Some measures may not be recognised as deliberately limiting people's freedom but still have that effect. Retaining mobility in later life is an important facet of well-being and independence. A variety of aids exist to help older people remain active, ranging from simple walking sticks, handrails and walking frames to specialised mechanisms that help patients lever themselves on to their feet. Patients with sight impairment need their spectacles or stick to find their way. Removal of such aids or leaving them out of reach in residential and in-patient settings can limit people's liberty and form an unacceptable measure of restraint. As is discussed in Chapter 2, removal of essential aids can also constitute negligence.

Maintaining mobility is particularly important as people age. Enforced immobility can have serious consequences for older people's health and quality of life. If not properly supported and supervised, older people's attempts to remain active can result in falls and fractures which are distressing and impinge on the quality of life. Care providers can have a difficult task to enable older people to keep mobile while minimising risks and ensuring the efficient running of the hospital ward, nursing home or care home. Nevertheless, there is a duty to try to promote mobility as part of the patient's overall care.

Protective measures: how they differ from 'restraint'

'Protective measures' sound reassuringly benign, whereas 'restraint' sounds more controversial. Although it would be useful to draw a clear distinction

The Ethics of Caring for Older People 2nd Edition. By British Medical Association.
Published 2009 by Blackwell Publishing Limited, ISBN: 9781405176279.

between them, in reality it is hard to do so and the borderline can be fluid. Despite the benign impression, protective measures can be unfairly or disproportionately restrictive of older people's activity. Bedrails, for example, are installed to protect people from accidentally falling out of bed and so can be categorised as a protective measure but they are a form of restraint if used deliberately to prevent people getting out of bed. An important distinction is that the aim of restraint (whether or not it is overt) is to restrict liberty, whereas protective measures are designed to manage risk without depriving individuals of their liberty. A deprivation of liberty without proper authority is unlawful. Although important for some patients, the routine use of measures such as bedrails for everyone reduces patients' independence and dignity. Older people are then unable to go to the toilet without assistance and risk soiling themselves or they fall from a greater height when climbing over. Health professionals have obligations to carry out appropriate risk assessments and minimise accidents, but the use of non-essential protective measures is controversial. However, some precautions must always be taken. For example, the Health and Safety Executive reports that bathwater temperatures for frail older people are not always checked and as a result numerous incidents of scalding, sometimes fatal, have occurred. Consequently, where communal bathrooms are used by at least one individual who is unable to judge the temperature of the bathwater, health and safety legislation requires that a mixer valve is fitted to the bath, set to 44°C. Even in the absence of such legislation, it is clear that some protective measures and common sense are essential in the provision of care to older people.

Electronic tagging, used to alert staff when a patient has wandered off the premises, is sometimes described as restraint but it is not necessarily so. It is a way of monitoring behaviour to which the response may be the use of restraint but it can also be a positive aid in alerting a member of staff to accompany and assist the patient. The intention of the care provider is a relevant factor in distinguishing between protective measures and restraint. Tagging and chair alarms which go off when people get up are protective measures if they are used to alert staff that assistance is needed, rather than to restrict movement. Tagging does not deprive people of their liberty, but it alerts staff about their movements.

Proportionality in the use of protective measures

Any method of restraint or protection needs to be carefully planned according to the circumstances of the case rather than being routine. The primary aim of some protective measures is to minimise falls by frail older people. This is important as falls are distressing and, even when no physical injury occurs, can lead to loss of confidence, increased in-patient stay in hospital and discharge into a nursing home. In an average 800-bed acute hospital trust, around 24 falls occur every week. Around 1% of falls in acute hospitals, community hospitals and mental health units result in fractures, compared to 5% of falls in the community[1]. The National Institute of Clinical Excellence recommends that all older people who come into contact with health professionals should be asked, as a matter of routine, whether they have fallen in the past year. Older people who report a fall, or are considered to be at risk of falling, should be offered interventions to improve strength and balance. Prevention of falls inevitably involves a risk/benefit analysis. Interventions to avoid any foreseeable harm need to be discussed with the individuals concerned and tailored to their needs. Protective measures are justified when they are proportionate to the harm to be avoided. This means looking at individuals' risks, discussing their wishes and recommending measures proportionate to the likelihood of harm and the seriousness of that harm.

Mentally competent older people

Like any other population group, older people are generally keen to preserve their health and avoid unnecessarily risky behaviour but they also need to assert their independence. If people have capacity, they are usually the best judges of their own interests and neither protective measures nor restraint should be used, unless they consent. Hospital patients and care home residents have the same rights as other people although some concessions may be required in communal settings to ensure the well-being of everyone. Any such concessions need to be understood by all and be proportionate to the situation. The right to freedom of movement is enshrined in the Human Rights Act 1998, which protects individuals from arbitrary restrictions on their liberty. Any form of restraint which restricts competent individuals' freedom, without their consent or some other overriding justification, could be a breach of the Act. An overriding justification could arise in cases where a competent person has to be restrained because their activities would cause harm to others. Competent patients have the right to risk their own health but are justifiably restrained if they represent a significant risk of harm to other people.

Older people who lack mental capacity

Some older people experience confusion, dementia or communication problems. Sometimes this results in high-risk or challenging behaviour. For older people who have impaired or fluctuating capacity, there are circumstances in which protective measures amounting to restraint are ethically and legally justified to protect themselves or other people. Health and care professionals need to strike a balance between preventing harm and preserving as much of individuals' independence of choice and movement as possible, without affecting other patients. When an individual lacks capacity, any decision affecting that person, including the use of protective measures and restraint, must be made on an assessment of their best interests. (Providing care in an individual's best interest is discussed in Chapter 4.) Assessment of people's best interests or of what would benefit them involves taking account of their known wishes and involving people close to them, including proxy decision-makers. In England and Wales, patients lacking external support should have an Independent Mental Capacity Advocate (IMCA)[2].

Older people with dementia can display aggression, inappropriate behaviour and wandering. Focussing on good communication and on the individual needs and circumstances in each case can defuse some problems. Aggressive behaviour is often the result of anxiety and fear in patients with cognitive impairment. Allowing them to wander in a safe manner, adjusting routines to suit their needs rather than imposing routines on them and exploring their preferences with regard to daily patterns can all reduce anxiety. Addressing the underlying causes of difficult behaviour and providing personalised support can reduce the need for protective measures that constitute restraint in many cases.

Case example – addressing the underlying causes of difficult behaviour

When S moved to a new care home, the record noted that she fought 'as if she were being raped' when the staff tried to help her use the toilet. She seemed not to understand what was going on and was frightened. In her previous nursing home, S had been regularly sedated so that the staff could take her to the toilet. Rather than use sedation as a means of restraint, the current staff decided to let S dictate the pattern of toileting. They did this by watching and taking their cue from her. They realised that S liked time and space to herself. Every afternoon, S was helped up to her room which was next door to the toilet and was able to manage going to the toilet herself. She drank well and kept dry. Later, however, as she began to fail physically, she lost the ability to go to the toilet herself. At that point, she allowed the staff, with whom she had built a relationship of trust, to provide her with pads and change her[3].

If patients' aggression or inappropriate behaviour poses a risk to other people, minimising the risks may well involve curtailing their freedom but the routine use of restraint, in the absence of appropriate risk assessment, is not acceptable nor in patients' best interests.

Tension between independence and protective measures

The use of protective measures and restraint should always be related to individuals' needs. Competent people should make their own decisions about whether they want protective measures. Restraint should not be imposed on them unless they represent a threat to the safety of others. Families may pressure staff to limit the risks their relatives take by imposing restrictive practices. Care providers need to make their own assessment, however, of whether restrictions are necessary and proportionate. Fear of complaints from relatives should not give rise to restrictions which are unnecessary and staff should explain why certain safeguards are not recommended in some cases. Decisions about restraint and protective measures are not always straightforward. A very real tension can arise between professionals' duty of care, which includes providing a safe environment, and the duty to encourage older people to retain their independence, which may involve risk. Assessment and discussion of each individual case is vital so that unnecessary restrictions can be avoided and patients' co-operation sought for those which are essential. All discussions and the resulting care plans should be carefully documented in patients' notes.

Risk management, protective measures and legal liability

Fear of incurring legal liability if accidents occur is one reason why care providers choose an excessively precautionary approach to risk management. Department of Health guidance[4] draws a distinction between putting people – especially those with impaired mental capacity – at risk and enabling competent people to take reasonable risks. People who are informed and have the mental capacity to choose can elect to live with a degree of risk. They are entitled to do so without it incurring any breach of duty of care by the professional or public authority but there needs to be open discussion with individuals about the consequences of their choices. Care providers could be exposed to litigation, however, if they place people in a position of risk that they have not chosen. There is an important distinction between doing this and enabling competent patients to take reasonable risks. The emphasis must be on supported decision-making and ensuring competent people have all the information they need to assess and interpret risks for themselves. In terms of managing legal liability, the Health Department's guidance stresses the importance of keeping accurate records of discussions about choice and risk. Such documentation is critical in order to protect people who are making choices, as well as the local authority or private care provider in the event of complaint or litigation.

Organisational pressures combined with shortage of staff can present difficult dilemmas when it comes to dealing with challenging or risky behaviour by patients. If there is a shortage of staff, it is easier to immobilise patients at risk of falling in low chairs rather than have staff available to help them to walk. Pressures to ensure the smooth running of health and care facilities are, however, unlikely to justify the restriction of the rights and freedoms of patients or residents.

Personalised care planning and alternatives to restricting liberty

Alternatives can be sought to the use of protective measures, including discussion with individuals and their relatives about other means of risk reduction. Personalised care planning helps identify what is important to individuals from their own perspective and helps ascertain how much restriction they are willing to tolerate. It encourages them to consider how their aims can be best achieved and what risks might be involved and can also be a way of overcoming the need for restrictive safeguards. Precautions to minimise any risk must be proportionate. A good example of a personalised approach can be seen in multi-factorial fall prevention programmes. Prevention of falls is one common reason for restricting the activity of older people as fall-related injuries are linked to a move to institutional care, overall reduction of physical activity and diminished quality of life. Multi-factorial fall prevention programmes are one way of addressing the risk, by providing individualised risk assessment and recommendations. Although as yet the evidence for their effectiveness remains limited[5], some evidence indicates that such interventions can reduce falls by up to 18%. Input in developing personalised recommendations is needed from a multidisciplinary team of doctors, nurses, psychiatrists, physiotherapists and occupational therapists.

Multi-factorial fall prevention programmes

- *Review medication associated with a risk of falls.*
- *Detect, treat or manage delirium, cardiovascular disease, incontinence, osteoporosis, eyesight problems.*
- *Recommend practical safeguards such as safer footwear.*
- *Improve balance by physiotherapy, exercise and access to walking aids.*
- *Review environmental factors such as flooring surface and pattern, lighting, design of doors and handrails, room layout, distance and spaces between hand holds, the line of sight for staff observing patients and trip hazards, including steps, clutter and cables[1].*

What is 'restraint'?

Restraint is often very similar to the use of protective measures. The distinction between the two is often just a matter of degree. Restraint involves restricting individuals' freedom to do things they want to do. It can be subtle or dramatic. Older people do not necessarily realise that low chairs and heavy doors are intended to keep them immobile. Building design can also serve to either restrict or facilitate movement by older people. Doors painted as bookcases, for example, and 'loop' layouts, which encourage people to walk in circles, are designed to distract people and prevent them from leaving buildings. Conversely, environmental design which is domestic, home-like and familiar to patients can be orientating and understandable. Removal of spectacles, walking frame or a stick can strongly deter people from moving around. Use of night clothes during waking hours or controlling language and behaviour by staff could all count as forms of unjustified restriction. Restraint can be overt, such as the use of straps on wheelchairs, or it can be covert and indirect such as doors that are difficult to open, furniture which makes walking with a frame impossible or the use of low furniture from which it is difficult to rise. Some of these measures may be barely noticed by older people but effectively limit their movement. The fact that people appear compliant and uncomplaining does not mean that their liberty is not unfairly restricted. More extreme and controversial methods of restraint include harnesses, locked doors, baffle locks and mittens. For people living with dementia, measures of restraint have included 'cocooning' them in sheets so that they cannot remove incontinence pads[6] and locking doors to restrict movement. If extreme or unwarranted measures are used, staff have an obligation to raise this with their supervisors and senior management. In some circumstances, it may be necessary to involve external bodies.

Categories of restraint

Physical – involves the use of physical force by one or more persons.

Mechanical – involves the use of equipment such as bedrails, mittens to stop patients removing nasogastric tubes or catheters.

Chemical – involving medication such as sedation.

Psychological – involves constantly telling people that some activity is forbidden, threatening force or threatening the removal of essential aids such as spectacles or walking sticks[7].

Restraint to prevent self-harm or harm to others

Health and care professionals have a common law right to use restraint to prevent harm to a person in their care or to another person. Restraint is permissible, for example, to prevent harm to a person who lacks capacity, as long as it is proportionate to the likelihood and seriousness of the harm. Restraint should involve the minimum amount of force for the shortest time possible. Problems arise, however, if the restraint results in 'deprivation of liberty' without appropriate safeguards. The common law does not justify actions which deprive individuals of their liberty and some other legal justification, such as the use of mental health legislation, is likely to be needed when patients are detained without their consent. Individuals can be restrained to prevent harm occurring but the response to any threat of violence must be reasonable and proportionate to the risk. Where there is a foreseeable need to manage violent patients, this should be planned for and staff trained in appropriate skills. Awareness of racial, cultural, social and gender differences can be important in understanding why individuals appear threatening and how the situation might be calmed. Staff should also have training in conflict avoidance and the safe use of restraints.

Case example – proportionate restraint

E lacked capacity as a result of dementia and was living in a residential care home. E sometimes mistook the dinner-bell for a bomb shelter alert and immediately tried to climb out of his bedroom window, not recognising any danger. The first time E attempted to climb out, he could not be verbally prevented through persuasion and was subsequently physically restrained. Under the circumstances, such restraint was the least harmful and restrictive measure possible. The action was proportionate to the aim which was to promote the patient's best interests by preventing the immediate risk until it had passed and longer-term safeguards could be considered. After a risk assessment, it was decided that, since E did not understand the danger of climbing out of the window, the window should be fitted with mechanical restrictions to limit the amount it could be opened. Whilst E's liberty was infringed to the extent that he was not free to fully open the window, the action was minimally restrictive and proportionate to the risk.

Chemical restraint and covert medication

A particularly controversial form of restraint is that involving medication. A parliamentary enquiry into elder abuse found that medication was 'in many cases, being used simply as a tool for the easier management of residents' rather than being in the patient's interests (Ref. [8], para 65). Organisations such as Action on Elder Abuse and the British Institute of Human Rights report the routine over-medication of older people in care homes, in order to keep them docile for staff convenience (Ref. [9], Ev 173 and Ev 222). There is also some evidence that a response to aggression in dementia sufferers is to prescribe powerful sedative drugs[9]. A 2001 study showed that 40% of older people with dementia in care homes were prescribed neuroleptic drugs, despite such medication being unlicensed for the routine treatment of dementia[10].

Covert medication breaches the principle of informed consent and so is unacceptable in the care and treatment of competent people. Staff should never mislead competent individuals about the purpose of their medication. Nor should they fail to answer their questions, on the grounds of lack of time or difficulties in communicating. Covert medication appears to be more common in residential care homes than in hospitals. Research suggests that over 70% of care homes have used covert medication[11].

Cases may arise in which covert medication is in the best interests of patients who lack mental capacity but it should not be routine. A decision to administer medication covertly to mentally incapacitated individuals should be taken by the clinician in overall charge of their medical care, in consultation with the multi-disciplinary care team. Changing the way medication is administered may also alter its benefits and risks. Crushing tablets, for example, may not be in line with the product license. Care providers may find it helpful to consult a pharmacist when assessing the risks associated with administering medication covertly. People close to incapacitated individuals should be involved in the decision. This includes proxy decision-makers and IMCAs where relevant (see Chapter 4). The reasons for a decision to give drugs covertly should be recorded in the patient's care plan and regularly reviewed. In making the decision, consideration should be given to:

- whether the patient genuinely lacks competence to consent or refuse treatment
- why covert medication is proposed and whether it is in the patient's best interests
- whether there are feasible alternatives that are more respectful of the individual's choice.

Case example – covert medication

J's dementia left him with fluctuating mental capacity. He had various other health problems, including a serious heart complaint which was effectively controlled by medication. When lucid, J understood the importance of continuing his medication and was particularly careful to take the drugs for his heart condition. In periods of confusion, however, J resisted any attempts by his wife to persuade him to take his medicine and said she was poisoning him. His GP thought that it would be best if another family member administered surreptitiously his heart medication on those occasions when J was reluctant to take it, as he risked a serious relapse or premature death without it. The fact that he accepted it willingly when lucid was seen as an indicator of his true preferences. When lucid, J could also consider giving advance authorisation for his medication to be administered covertly during periods of confusion. In doing so, J would have the opportunity to exercise a maximum amount of choice despite his dementia.

Principles concerning use of restraint

Patient consent

There is seldom a justification for using restraint on competent older people, other than in exceptional cases where they pose a risk of harm to others. Concerns about institutional liability may need to be investigated by taking legal advice if competent people refuse to comply with health and safety measures. Discussion of the risks and explanation of why safeguards are recommended may gain the individual's agreement to them. If a competent person agrees to a restriction, it is not restraint. To the degree to which they are capable, patients with impaired capacity should also be involved in decisions about how restrictions are applied. Even if they lack the capacity to consent to the use of protective measures or restraint, they are more likely to accept them if they can understand why they are proposed. If restraint distresses an incapacitated patient, alternatives should be explored and discussed with people close to the patient and any proxy decision-maker.

Individualised risk assessment

Restrictions must be proportionate, based on a personalised risk assessment and never used routinely. A risk assessment on admission to hospital or a residential setting is a crucial part of care planning. In many instances, disruptive or risky behaviour can be mitigated through gaining an understanding of the cause of it. Unsettled or disruptive behaviour may be a result of unmet needs or poor ability to communicate[6]. If the triggers of disruptive behaviour are understood, they are easier to address without resorting to restraint. Much work has been done, for example, involving older people who wander. Emphasis is placed on looking at the underlying reasons for the wandering. Once triggers and motivations are understood, personalised care can be implemented.

Least restrictive alternative

A House of Commons Select Committee enquiry in 2004 indicated that restraint is used in health and care settings when other, less restrictive measures, would be more suitable[8]. Rather than preventing patients walking around when at risk of falling, encouraging them to ring a bell for assistance and giving them a set of recommendations about how to help them avoid risk may work better. Tagging is often suggested as an alternative to restraint. Rather than locking doors, staff can be alerted when 'at risk' patients cross certain boundaries. Those individuals can then either be monitored or accompanied, depending on their agreed care plan. When restraint is unavoidable, it should be the least restrictive option, for the minimum amount of time. Freedoms can be restricted but only in a manner proportionate to the harm the restrictions are intended to prevent.

Care planning, review and communication

Multidisciplinary care planning can minimise the need for restraint. As is discussed in Chapter 2, good communication between staff is a crucial facet of patient care. Unless individuals are assessed as requiring bedrails, for example, this method of protection should not be routinely used simply because beds are fitted with them. In order to avoid routine use becoming the norm, individualised discussion needs to take place about how to protect or restrain patients.

Record-keeping

Record-keeping of discussions with patients and care home residents is an important facet of care. Except for emergency situations, decisions about the use of restrictive measures should be made in advance and the reasons for it recorded in the care plan. This should specify in what circumstances restraint may be used, what form it will take and how often it will be reviewed. Every episode of restraint should be fully documented and regularly reviewed. A record should also be made of discussions with individuals about their preferences in risk management. Such records assume particular importance in the event of complaint or litigation. They are also an important point of reference for members of the healthcare team so that they all know what has been agreed for an individual's care.

'Bournewood safeguards' – restriction and deprivation of liberty

Restraint should only involve a specific, time-limited restriction of individual freedom but there is a risk it could develop into a more systematic form of control that could amount to 'deprivation of liberty'. If people are to be deprived of their liberty, there must be some lawful justification and some safeguards. For patients with a mental illness, use of mental health legislation should be considered if the patients meet the statutory requirements. Mental health legislation would constitute a legal justification for their deprivation of liberty, with appropriate safeguards and an appeals mechanism.

The 'Bournewood' case, which was heard by the European Court of Human Rights[12], dealt with complex issues and set some standards about what constitutes an unlawful deprivation of liberty. These standards are referred to as 'Bournewood safeguards'. The facts of the case are set out in the following box. The judgement marked a significant step forward in the recognition of the rights of incompetent individuals. It led to increased legal awareness of the rights of older people with impaired capacity.

The Bournewood case

HL, an autistic man with severe learning disabilities, was informally admitted to Bournewood Hospital under the common law rather than under mental health legislation. Whilst HL was compliant in the treatment, it was clear that he did not have the capacity to consent to it. He was subject to continuous supervision and was not free to leave the hospital. The European Court of Human Rights found that he had been deprived of his liberty unlawfully, violating Articles 5(1) and 5(4) of the European Convention on Human Rights, even though the English law tests of 'best interests' and 'necessity' had been satisfied. HL had been detained without a legal procedure (i.e. not under the provisions of the Mental Health Act) and without procedural safeguards. He did not have rapid access to a court or tribunal. Detention without such safeguards was deemed a failure to protect individuals against arbitrary deprivations of liberty. The Court made clear that the question of whether someone has, in fact, been deprived of liberty depends on the particular circumstances of the case and that the difference between deprivation and restriction of liberty was said to be one of degree and intensity.

HL v United Kingdom[12]

Many patients who lack full capacity but are compliant in restrictions on their liberty are older people. Patients with dementia or other cognitive illnesses, for example, are prevented from leaving residential care homes and comply with that restriction. The European Court judgement highlighted the importance of providing care in ways that, as far as possible, avoid any actual deprivation of liberty. Where deprivation of liberty is unavoidable – that is to say it is necessary, proportionate and in the individual's best interests – it can be permissible, provided appropriate safeguards are followed. The legal interpretation of what constitutes 'deprivation of liberty' is not clearly defined but it is likely to cover situations in which complete control is exercised over the individual. Health and care professionals need to know how to recognise a potential deprivation of liberty, how to identify ways of providing care that can avoid it and the safeguards that must be implemented should it prove unavoidable. These safeguards only apply to individuals who lack the mental capacity to consent to the arrangements made for their care and are looked after in circumstances that amount to a deprivation of liberty. Treatment of these individuals is regulated by mental capacity legislation. The Bournewood safeguards apply irrespective of whether the deprivation of liberty takes place in a public or a private institution.

Identifying deprivation of liberty

Whilst the implications of Bournewood are wide ranging, their impact on practice is hard to gauge. A particularly difficult issue for health and care professionals is that there is not a definitive legal account of what 'deprivation of liberty' entails. Until the safeguards have been in force for a period and the limits tested in court, some ambiguity as to what constitutes deprivation of liberty is likely to remain. In its judgment the European Court stated that 'the key factor ... is that the healthcare professionals treating and managing the applicant exercised complete and effective control over his care and movements' and that 'the applicant was under continuous supervision and control and was not free to leave'. In everyday terms, problems will arise in identifying when a patient's aimless but potentially dangerous wandering becomes an intention to leave and therefore when restricting such a patient's movement becomes unlawful.

What constitutes 'deprivation of liberty'?

The Court gave some directions on what would contribute to deprivation of an individual's liberty:

- *use of restraint or sedation to admit a person who is resisting;*
- *professionals exercising complete control over care and movement for a significant period;*

- *professionals controlling assessments, treatment, contacts and residence;*
- *individual prevented from leaving if he/she attempted to do so (by either force or threat of force);*
- *request by other carers for the person to be discharged to their care refused;*
- *individual unable to maintain social contacts since restrictions placed on access to other people;*
- *individual loses autonomy because he/she is under continuous supervision and control[13].*

The Court stated that the difference between restriction and deprivation of liberty is one of degree and intensity, rather than the type of restrictive measures involved. Although cases have to be assessed individually, it is likely that any systematic and complete control over an individual in care would count as deprivation of liberty. This differs from restraint and restriction of liberty which are situation- or time-specific. Deprivation of liberty is much more likely where individual movement is systematically controlled. The use of locked doors and other barriers which stop people moving freely are likely to constitute a deprivation of liberty. The ethical principles engaged in assessing whether the deprivation of liberty is justified are the same principles engaged in the assessment of any other degree of restrictive measure.

Avoiding deprivation of liberty

The law and best practice emphasise that all individuals should be treated in ways that restrict their freedom as little as possible. Decisions made on behalf of individuals who lack mental capacity must be the least restrictive of the available options. Wherever possible, deprivation of liberty should be avoided. Active measures should be taken by health and care professionals to avoid any unnecessary restrictions, and decision-making should involve, as fully as possible, both the individuals and those who are close to them. Some good practice guidance is available in relation to avoiding deprivation of liberty.

Practical measures for avoiding 'deprivation of liberty'

- *Decisions should be taken and reviewed in a structured way and the reasons behind them recorded.*
- *Effective documented care planning, which could include, where appropriate, the Care Programme approach, Single Assessment Process, Person-Centred Planning*

> or Unified Assessment. This should include appropriate and documented involvement of family, friends, carers or other people interested in the individual's welfare.
> - A proper documented assessment of the individual's capacity to decide whether to consent to the care being proposed is of key importance.
> - Alternatives to admission to hospital or residential care should be carefully considered and any restrictions placed on liberty in care homes or hospitals should be kept to the minimum necessary.
> - Appropriate information, presented in ways that are sensitive to individual needs, should be offered to patients and those involved in their care.
> - Where appropriate, local advocacy services should be enrolled to provide support to patients and their families, friends and carers. IMCAs must be involved in certain circumstances – see Chapter 4.
> - Care should be taken to ensure that patients remain in contact with people close to them.
> - The assessment of patients' capacity, and their care plan, should be kept under review.

Authorising deprivation of liberty – England and Wales

When an incapacitated patient is identified as being at risk of deprivation of liberty in a hospital or care home, the 'managing authority' of that hospital or home has to make an application to a 'supervisory body' to request an authorisation. In the case of an NHS hospital, the managing authority is the NHS body responsible for its running. In the case of a private hospital or care home, the managing authority is the person registered under Part 2 of the Care Standards Act 2000. If the patient is in hospital, the supervisory body in England is the Primary Care Trust (PCT). In Wales, it is the National Assembly for Wales, unless the PCT has commissioned the relevant care, in which case the PCT will be the supervisory body. In both England and Wales, if the patient is in a care home the supervisory body is the local authority. The application for supervision should be made in advance, except in urgent situations when the care home or hospital can issue an emergency authorisation, ensuring that the decision is documented and seek a standard authorisation within 7 days.

Once a person is identified as potentially being deprived of liberty, the hospital or care home must establish whether there is someone (who is not providing care or treatment in a professional or paid capacity) who could appropriately look after the incapacitated person's interests. This could be a relative or someone close to the patient. If it is not possible to identify such an individual, the supervisory body must instruct an IMCA to represent the patient. (IMCAs are discussed in Chapter 4.) This person's role is to maintain contact with the individual and provide representation and support. Once the application has been made, the authorising authority assesses the individual to verify that he or she is being deprived of liberty and that it is lawful.

The assessment process is laid out in six separate sections

Age – the person must be over 18.

Mental health – the person must be suffering from a mental disorder within the meaning of the Mental Health Act 1983 (as amended), ignoring the exemption for people with learning disabilities. This means that the learning disability does not have to be associated with abnormally aggressive or seriously irresponsible conduct.

Mental capacity – the person must lack capacity in relation to the decision about whether or not they should stay in the hospital or care home for the purpose of being given care or treatment.

Best interests – the purpose of this is to establish whether deprivation of liberty is occurring and, if so, whether it is in individuals' best interests in order to prevent harm to themselves and whether deprivation is proportionate to the risks.

Eligibility – this relates to the individual's status under the Mental Health Act 1983 (as amended). If a person is detained under the Mental Health Act 1983, they are not eligible.

No refusals – this is to ensure that the authorisation would not conflict with another authority, such as an advance refusal or a decision made by someone authorised under a Lasting Power of Attorney (this is discussed in Chapter 4).

Who can undertake a Bournewood assessment?

Regulations specify that anybody that the supervisory body considers to have the necessary skills and experience can undertake the assessments. There must be a minimum of two assessors. Assessment of mental health and that of 'best interests' must be made by different people. While the best interests assessor may be employed by the supervisory body or managing authority, he or she cannot be involved in the care of the person or in decisions about the person's care. If the individual is in a care home, the assessor cannot be on the staff of the care home. None of the assessors can have a personal financial interest in the care of the person they are assessing. In addition, the assessor cannot be related to the person being assessed or to a person with a personal financial interest in the person's care.

Northern Ireland

At the time of writing there are no formal provisions in primary legislation for the treatment of 'Bournewood' patients in Northern Ireland. The Northern Irish government intends to make such provisions under forthcoming mental capacity legislation. As soon as possible after the enactment of such legislation, guidance will be provided on the website of the British Medical Association. Until such legislation has been issued, professionals caring for incapacitated patients who are informally deprived of their liberty should seek legal advice on a case-by-case basis.

Scotland

In Scotland, the appropriate actions to be taken if a person is deemed to be deprived of his or her liberty are governed by the Mental Health (Care and Treatment) (Scotland) Act 2003 and the Adults with Incapacity (Scotland) Act 2000. If a patient is in hospital and remains informally detained, there is a procedure for this to be appealed to the Mental Health Tribunal for Scotland under mental health legislation. Anyone with an interest in the patient's welfare, including paid carers, can apply to the Tribunal for a decision as to whether the patient is being unlawfully detained. Unlike England and Wales, however, there are no statutory mechanisms for ensuring oversight of isolated individuals who are un-befriended. Professionals caring for incapacitated patients who are informally deprived of their liberty should seek legal advice on a case-by-case basis.

Adults who are deprived of their liberty in residential care homes should have the oversight of a welfare guardian under the terms of the Adults with Incapacity (Scotland) Act. This involves an application to the Sheriff (see Chapter 4). Anyone with an interest in the individual can apply to the Sheriff, but the local authority is obliged to do so if no one applies on behalf of the patient.

Summary of chapter

- *Each older individual should have a personalised risk assessment and care plan.*
- *Competent older people should participate in decisions if protective measures are recommended for them and should not be subject to compulsion or covert measures. They should participate in discussions on how they can safeguard their own health and minimise their risk of accidents.*
- *People can be justifiably restrained if their behaviour poses a risk of serious harm to others.*

- For people with impaired mental capacity, protective measures should restrict their freedom of movement as little as possible while providing them with a safe environment. Any deprivation of liberty without proper authority is unlawful.
- Methods of restraint – direct or indirect – should not be used as an alternative to adequate staffing levels.
- Restraint must be planned, discussed, documented and proportionate to the risks.

References

1. NHS National Patient Safety Agency (2007). *Slips, Trips and Falls in Hospital. The Third Report from the Patient Safety Observatory.* NPSA, London.
2. This is discussed in detail in Chapter 4.
3. This case example is based on one given by Chester R (1998). *Towards Continence: Approaches to Continence in Homes for Older People.* Counsel and Care, London.
4. Department of Health (2007). *Independence, Choice and Risk: A Guide to Best Practice in Supported Decision Making.* DH, London. This guidance is aimed at social care professionals but is also applicable to health professionals working in multidisciplinary teams.
5. Gates S, Fisher JD, Cooke MW, et al. (2008). Multifactorial assessment and targeted intervention for preventing falls and injuries among older people in community and emergency care settings: systematic review and meta-analysis. *Br Med J* **336:** 130–3.
6. Commission for Social Care Inspection (2007). *Rights, Risks and Restraints. An Exploration into the Use of Restraint in the Care of Older People.* CSCI, London.
7. Royal College of Nursing (2008). *Let's Talk About Restraint – Rights, Risks and Responsibility.* RCN, London.
8. House of Commons Health Committee (2004). *Elder Abuse Second Report of Session 2003–04. Volume 1.* The Stationery Office Ltd, London.
9. Joint Committee on Human Rights (2007). *The Human Rights of Older People in Healthcare. Eighteenth Report of Session 2006–07. Volume 2 – Oral and Written Evidence.* The Stationery Office, London.
10. Margallo-Lana M, Swan A, O'Brian J, et al. (2001). Management of behavioural and psychiatric symptoms amongst dementia sufferers living in care environment. *Int J Geriatr Psychiatry* **16:** 39–44.
11. Mental Welfare Commission for Scotland (2006). *Covert Medication. Legal and Practical Guidance.* Mental Welfare Commission for Scotland, Edinburgh.
12. HL v United Kingdom (2004) 40 EHRR 761.
13. Department of Health (2006). *The Bournewood Safeguards: Draft Illustrative Code of Practice.* DH, London, para 25. Further information on the new code is awaited following consultations which ended in January 2008.

Further resources

Commission for Social Care Inspection (2007). *Rights, Risks and Restraints. An Exploration into the Use of Restraint in the Care of Older People.* CSCI, London.

Counsel and Care UK (2002). *Showing Restraint: Challenging the Use of Restraint in Care Homes.* Counsel and Care, London.

Mental Welfare Commission for Scotland (2006). *Covert Medication: Legal and Practical Guidance.* MWCS, Edinburgh.

Mental Welfare Commission for Scotland (2006). *Rights, Risks and Limits to Freedom. Principles and Good Practice for Practitioners Considering Restraint in Residential Care Settings.* MWCS, Edinburgh.

National Institute of Clinical Excellence (2005). *Violence: The Short-Term Management of Disturbed/Violent Behaviour in In-patient Psychiatric Settings and Emergency Departments.* NICE, London.

Royal College of Nursing (2008). *Let's Talk About Restraint – Rights, Risks and Responsibility.* RCN, London.

Chapter 7 Helping people make decisions in advance

Planning for future contingencies

As medical technology advances, it will become increasingly possible to detect in advance some medical conditions that may later render patients incapable of deciding for themselves or of communicating their wishes. Blood tests are being developed, for example, to identify early signs of conditions such as Alzheimer's disease which previously could only be diagnosed once patients showed symptoms of the condition. Not everyone would want to have such information in advance, but a reliable blood test would give those who do an opportunity to prepare and make decisions about their future care. Some people fear that, if they become mentally incapable, they will be given medical interventions they do not want or not be given treatments they do want. The purpose of advance decisions is to provide for choices that may need to be made in the future, when the individual will no longer be able to express a view.

Advance decision-making can be useful for individuals who have strong views, a medical condition likely to involve a future period of mental impairment and predictable treatment options. It is not necessarily right for everybody. Some older people make clear that they do not want to know the full implications of their diagnosis but prefer to have decisions made for them by people they trust. Appointing someone to do this is discussed in detail in Chapter 4. In this chapter, we look principally at formal advance decisions to refuse treatment (ADRT). Apart from mental health interventions covered by statute, competent adults can lawfully refuse medical procedures contemporaneously or in advance. If they meet certain criteria, advance refusals are legally binding on health care providers. There are various reasons why people think they need to make plans in advance about how their care should be handled at the end of life. One common reason, flagged up in 2006 by focus groups involving older people and co-ordinated by Help the Aged, was the reluctance of patients' relatives to discuss with them what will happen at the end of their lives. Their families'

The Ethics of Caring for Older People 2nd Edition. By British Medical Association.
Published 2009 by Blackwell Publishing Limited, ISBN: 9781405176279.

attempts to avoid such matters in advance made some older people worried that, if they did not write down their wishes, the wrong choices would be made for them[1].

What is an advance decision?

Adults who understand the implications of their choices can state in advance how they wish to be treated if they later suffer loss of mental capacity. General statements they make may be helpful in assessing their best interests later but are not necessarily legally binding. Nor are requests for future treatment legally binding in the same way that informed refusals are. Any advance decision is always superseded by a competent contemporaneous decision by the individual concerned or by the decision of a proxy decision-maker who was subsequently appointed to make that decision.

Various terms are used to describe methods for making decisions or indicating preferences in advance. These include 'advance decisions', 'living wills' and 'advance statements'. Such choices can be recorded in a written document, a clear oral statement, a signed printed card, a smart card or a note of a discussion recorded in the patient's file. Any of these may convey a sense of the individual's wishes but, to be legally binding, an advance refusal of treatment must fit the criteria set out later.

An advance decision is a clear instruction of refusing a medical proce-dure or intervention such as participation in research. Voluntarily made by a competent and informed adult, an unambiguous advance decision to refuse treatment is likely to have legal force. Health professionals are gener-ally bound to comply when the refusal specifically addresses the situation which has arisen.

An advance authorisation or request reflects the individual's preferences for certain positive interventions after capacity is lost. Like advance refusals, advance requests and authorisations must be made when the individual has capacity and is aware of the implications. Requests for help identify how people would like to be treated but are not binding, if in conflict with professional judgement. Nevertheless, in some circumstances, the health team may be obliged to provide artificial nutrition and hydration (ANH) at the end of life if it is clear that this is what the patient wanted. The legal situation regarding advance requests for ANH is complex. It is summarised below but it is also advisable to consult specialised guidance[2].

Although health professionals are most commonly confronted by advance decisions in relation to medical treatment, patients can also express other wishes in this way which should be respected.

Case example – advance refusal of family contact

P was admitted for hospice care when approaching the end of his life. He had been married several times but only remained on good terms with the children of his last marriage. The hospice was contacted by his son from a previous relationship who was keen to see him but P was adamant in refusing the visit. The hospice staff hoped he would relent and feared it would be psychologically damaging for the son, who had not seen him for many years, not to have some final contact but P remained intransigent. He willingly received visits from his more recent family. In his final days, P was unconscious and his son renewed his requests to at least have a last sight of his father, which he thought would provide a sense of closure. Although it seemed harsh, the hospice staff were obliged to respect P's wishes, as he had made them very clear. It would have breached his wishes to permit his son to have access to P, even after the father had lost consciousness and it would have upset the rest of the family who were well aware of P's views and respected them, even if they did not agree with them.

Do-not-attempt-resuscitation decisions

One form of advance decision that often involves discussion with patients but is normally made by clinicians rather than by patients themselves is a do-not-attempt-resuscitation (DNAR) decision. This states that cardiopulmonary resuscitation (CPR) should not be attempted for a particular patient in the event of cardiac arrest. DNAR decisions are mentioned here as they represent one facet of advance decision-making. CPR is discussed in more detail in Chapter 8, where it is made clear that, despite what the public often assumes, CPR is frequently unsuccessful in restoring heart function and breathing. It also has significant risks, including fractured bones, brain damage, ruptured internal organs or that death occurs in an undignified or traumatic manner.

A DNAR decision may be appropriate if:

- *a competent, informed patient has refused CPR in advance;*
- *the healthcare team is as certain as it can be that attempting CPR would not restart this patient's heart and breathing, and the patient would not gain any benefit from the procedure being attempted;*
- *there would be no benefit for the patient, for whom only a very brief extension of life could be achieved as other underlying illnesses mean that death cannot be averted, even if resuscitation were successful;*

> • the expected benefits – if CPR were successful – would still be outweighed by
> the burdens for the patient because, for example, he or she is likely to be left
> mentally incapacitated, severely physically disabled and in pain.

Patients who wish to refuse CPR need to either make an advance decision to that effect or ensure that their clinician has made a DNAR decision for them. If the health care team consider resuscitation should not be attempted, it needs to be communicated sensitively to the patient, those close to the patient and other professionals providing care. It also needs to be recorded in the patient's notes. Detailed guidance on decisions relating to CPR has been published by the British Medical Association, Royal College of Nursing and Resuscitation Council (see 'Further resources' at the end of this chapter).

Legal position on advance refusals of treatment

In England and Wales, ADRT are covered by the Mental Capacity Act 2005 which came into force in October 2007. In Scotland, the Adults with Incapacity (Scotland) Act 2000 came into force in 2002 and introduced a statutory framework for the medical treatment of incapacitated adults. Although it does not specifically cover advance decisions, it obliges health professionals to take into account the patient's past and present wishes, however communicated. In Northern Ireland, there is no statute on this subject, but English case law, which sets out criteria for ADRT, is likely to be followed.

Mental capacity needed to make an advance refusal of medical treatment

As is discussed in Chapter 4, different levels of mental capacity are required for different types of decision, depending on the implications of the choice to be made. The level of capacity required to request or refuse treatment in advance is the same level that would be required for making the decision contemporaneously. Mental capacity can be demonstrated by patients who lack insight into other aspects of their life as long as they understand the implications of the specific choice before them. In 1993, for example, the courts[3] upheld the rights of a patient with a psychotic disorder to refuse validly in advance the amputation of his gangrenous foot even though he held demonstrably erroneous views on some other matters. But even clear and specific ADRT cannot override other legislation. Thus, an ADRT cannot override the legal authority to give compulsory treatment under mental health legislation.

Legal criteria in England and Wales

In order for an ADRT to be legally binding on the health care team, certain criteria set out in the Mental Capacity Act 2005 must be met. If advance decisions do not meet these criteria, they can still be useful in assessing the patient's best interests but are not legally binding. In order to be legally binding, an ADRT must be valid and applicable and authority to make the same decision must not have been subsequently transferred to a person with lasting power of attorney (see Chapter 4).

Criteria for a valid ADRT

- *The person making it was a competent, informed adult when it was made.*
- *The refusal has not been withdrawn.*
- *No attorney has been appointed later to make the decision.*
- *There is no indication that the person changed his/her mind.*
- *The decision specifies – in medical or lay terms – the treatment refused.*
- *The circumstances that have arisen are those envisaged in the decision.*
- *The individual lacks capacity to make decisions when the refusal is implemented.*
- *If the refusal is likely to result in the person's death, the person recognised that and indicated that it is to apply even if death will predictably result.*
- *The decision is in writing.*
- *It is signed and witnessed.*
- *If doubt exists about the validity of an advance refusal of treatment, the Court of Protection decides.*

Legal criteria in Scotland

ADRT are not covered by statute in Scotland and nor have there been any specific cases considered by the courts there. The Code of Practice issued under the Adults with Incapacity (Scotland) Act advises that a competently made advance decision should be seen as a strong indication of the patient's former wishes. Health professionals are obliged to take account of such known former wishes and are likely to be bound by a valid advance refusal of treatment although this has not been tested in the Scottish courts. If a case were brought, it is likely that Scottish courts would take a similar approach to the English courts. Prior to the passing of the Mental Capacity Act in England and Wales, a number of English legal cases had already established that a valid advance refusal of treatment has the same legal authority as a contemporaneous refusal[4]. In certain cases, respecting the advance refusal of competent adult patients is also likely to be seen as a requirement of Articles 5 and 8 of the Human Rights Act.

Legal criteria in Northern Ireland

There is no statute in Northern Ireland either and so the common law about respecting patients' advance wishes applies there. English legal cases constituted the common law position in England until the Mental Capacity Act and they remain the basis of the common law in Northern Ireland.

Common law criteria for validity of an advance refusal of treatment

- *The person making it was a competent adult when it was made.*
- *The patient had sufficient, accurate information to make a valid decision.*
- *There is nothing to indicate the individual changed his/her mind.*
- *The circumstances that have arisen are those that were envisaged by the individual.*
- *The patient was not subjected to undue influence in making the decision.*

Advance refusal of essential nursing care

Organisations such as the British Medical Association do not consider that people should be able to refuse basic nursing care in advance. Sometimes termed 'basic care', essential nursing care covers the activities primarily intended to keep patients comfortable rather than to extend their lives. It is unlikely that people would want to refuse procedures designed to alleviate their pain, symptoms or distress. Nor would most people decline things such as help with feeding themselves when their mental capacity is lost. Most health bodies think it is unacceptable and contrary to good practice for health professionals to leave a person, who is now lacking capacity, in pain or discomfort even if there appears to be an advance refusal to that effect. Such an advance refusal would need to be challenged. It may be that the individual had not been properly informed or was unable to envisage the consequences of the choice and legal advice may be required. The courts have made clear, however, that artificial feeding and hydration are not part of essential care but are procedures that patients can refuse or which may not be offered if deemed futile. The concept of a fundamental level of care, which should not be refused or withdrawn, is also mentioned in Chapter 8.

Emergencies when it is unknown if a refusal exists

As a general principle, the law expects health professionals to act reasonably in the circumstances in which they find themselves. In an emergency situation, where it is unclear whether an unconscious or mentally impaired patient has refused treatment in advance, it is reasonable not to delay medical care if that would result in a serious risk to the person's life or health. If there is a valid and applicable advance refusal of treatment, it should be followed. If treatment has been initiated in good faith and an advance decision is subsequently discovered which is clearly relevant to the current circumstances and fulfils the criteria for validity and applicability, it should be followed.

Dilemmas arise when older patients with a serious diagnosis have not envisaged a more unpredictable event such as a traffic accident, when making their advance refusal of treatment. Their refusal of life-prolonging treatment was probably never intended to apply to a situation in which recovery of their mental faculties is a possibility. If their intention is clearly spelled out, it should be evident that the advance refusal is not applicable to the current situation. If, however, it is unclear whether the individual intended an advance decision to apply in all circumstances of impaired capacity, including an apparently unforeseen situation, the advice about assessing validity and applicability should be followed.

Advance requests for treatment

When they have a diagnosis likely to involve loss of mental capacity, it is good practice to offer patients the opportunity to talk about foreseeable future treatment options, if they want to discuss them. Some are keen to prepare themselves. Not everyone, however, wants to talk about the future, and so it is important that care providers do not lose sight of the importance of patients' willingness to do so. It is also important not to generate unrealistic expectations about treatments that might be available. General advance care planning is discussed in more detail in Chapter 8. If there has been no advance discussion prior to the individual losing mental capacity, health professionals are obliged to act on the basis of their assessment of what would be in that person's best interests. (This is discussed in detail in Chapters 3 and 4.) Discussion and advance decision-making can be helpful if competent people have a diagnosis likely to involve later mental impairment and have clear views which are unlike those of most other patients. Although they can request a particular treatment now or in the future, it does not mean it will automatically be provided. Doctors cannot be obliged to provide clinically inappropriate procedures or treatments which have a small chance of success. If the requested intervention cannot achieve its physiological aim, or if its burdens outweigh the benefits for the particular individual, it will not be provided. Nor can treatment automatically be provided if it would deprive other people of opportunities for medical care when resources are limited.

Legal position on advance requests

In terms of life-prolonging interventions, health professionals have a legal as well as an ethical duty to protect life, under Article 2 of the European Human Rights Convention, but its scope is limited. Basically, life does not have to be prolonged at all costs, but various factors, such as the individual's known wishes and the likelihood of treatment succeeding, need to be considered. In some circumstances, advance requests for specific life-prolonging treatment such as ANH should be respected. The law in this area is complex and so it is advisable to consult legal advice or expert guidance for those situations[2]. The Burke case (below) clarified that doctors have a duty to take reasonable steps to comply with patients' requests that ANH be provided in future.

Legal case – Burke v GMC

Mr Burke was a 45-year-old man who suffered from cerebellar ataxia with peripheral neuropathy, a progressively degenerative condition that follows a similar course to multiple sclerosis. It was foreseeable that as his condition worsened, he would lose the ability to swallow. He would then need ANH. Medical evidence indicated that he would retain mental capacity until close to his death and so would be able to make his wishes known. Mr Burke worried, however, that if he lost his mental capacity, his former wishes would be ignored. Doctors treating him would be governed by the guidance on withdrawing life-prolonging treatment issued by the regulatory body, the General Medical Council. This gave doctors the discretion to withdraw ANH even if a person's death was not imminent. Mr Burke claimed that the guidance was incompatible with Articles 2, 3, 6, 8 and 14 of the European Convention on Human Rights. In July 2004, a judge agreed with him but this judgment was later overturned by the Court of Appeal. Even though it contradicted the earlier ruling, the Appeal Court said that there was no question of ANH being withdrawn because Mr Burke had made clear that he wanted it when he was no longer able to express his wishes. The Appeal Court ruled that doctors' duty of care included the obligation to take reasonable steps to prolong

> the patient's life where that was the patient's wish. To deliberately interrupt life-prolonging treatment, in the face of a competent patient's previously expressed wish to be kept alive, with the intention of thereby terminating the patient's life would leave the doctor with no answer to a charge of murder.
>
> *R (on the application of Burke) v GMC[5]*

The duty to provide life-prolonging treatment, where this is the patient's wish, does not extend to treatment that doctors believe is not clinically indicated. What is reasonable in each situation needs to be judged in the context of each case.

Practicalities in relation to drawing up ADRT

There are some practical issues that need to be considered by individuals who want to draft ADRT. Practical questions also arise for health professionals caring for them or later implementing the patient's decisions. If they have strong views, patients need to consider how to make those clearly known. Various steps are open to them. Some draw up a clear statement of the treatment to be refused that is lodged with their medical record. Some carry copies with them or a card indicating that they refuse certain procedures. Jehovah's Witnesses, for example, often carry cards stating their refusal of blood products. In addition to specific ADRT, ongoing discussion about how patients' general wishes about future care and treatment may be recorded on the summary care record, developed as part of the NHS Connecting for Health Care Records Service project.

One of the most important steps that people can take to ensure that their wishes and values are respected later is to discuss them with their families. Dilemmas can arise when relatives are unsure or disagree among themselves about what the now incapacitated person would have wanted.

Provision of information

Ideally, advance decisions should be drafted following discussion with health professionals rather than in isolation. Medical advice can lead to a better-informed declaration but it is important for any adviser to help patients clarify their own wishes rather than influence them. The main purpose of advance planning is for patients to try and control as much as they can, things that are likely to happen to them later when they are no longer mentally competent. It is important, however, that they do not have unrealistic expectations about the extent to which the end of anyone's life can be controlled and managed as they would want. This is discussed further in Chapter 8. Foreseeable options and uncertainties need to be explained and it is important to be both sensitive and frank. The professionals who may subsequently have to implement patients' advance decisions will rely on the fact that the individual was properly informed when formulating them.

Verbal advance decisions and verbal amendments

Individuals suffering from a condition requiring long-term care have opportunities for discussion with the health care team over a long period. They may feel their wishes are sufficiently well known, or reflected in the notes, so that there is no need to write them down. In hospice or specialist palliative care settings, this form of oral advance discussion is common practice. A general expression of views cannot be accorded the same weight as a firm decision but can be helpful in illustrating the patient's known wishes, even if expressed in a verbal form that would not meet the legal criteria. Nevertheless, there are advantages to recording firm decisions in a written document. Many older patients only lose capacity relatively shortly before death. Until the point that capacity is lost, the individual's current views will always outweigh anything he or she decided earlier. Individuals can verbally amend or withdraw their advance decision at any time, as long as they retain capacity.

Written advance decisions

Written ADRT should use clear language and be signed by the individual and a witness. Although not legally binding, statements of future preferences for care and treatment can assist health professionals to accommodate decisions which are so personal that only the individual concerned could make them. A key concern for many people is to be able to say where they would like to be cared for and where they wish to die or whom they want called to their bedside. People cannot authorise or refuse in advance, procedures which they could not authorise or refuse contemporaneously. They cannot authorise unlawful procedures, such as assisted dying, nor insist upon futile or inappropriate treatment. If individuals want to refuse life-sustaining treatment, they need to say clearly in the advance decision that they are aware that this refusal is likely to result in their death. In England and Wales, this is a legal requirement for validity under the Mental Capacity Act 2005 and such clarity of intention is also advisable in Scotland and Northern Ireland where there is no statute covering this point.

Health professionals witnessing advance decisions

Health professionals are often asked to witness an ADRT or note the patient's advance wishes in the health record. If they do so, it may be assumed that they verified the patient's capacity when the decision was made or the preferences given. Arguably, however, this should not be automatically assumed, given that doctors do not normally assess patients' mental capacity unless there are reasons to question it. Adults are assumed to have mental capacity unless there is evidence to the contrary. Health professionals who act as a witness and have no reason to believe that the patient suffers from impaired capacity may add a note to that effect. If, however, there is any reason to doubt that the patient understands the implications of the decision, and especially if the consequences of the decision are likely to be serious or clearly pejorative for the individual, an assessment of capacity is advisable. Assessment of capacity is discussed in Chapter 3.

Reviewing advance decisions

In England and Wales, the question sometimes arises as to whether an ADRT drafted long before the Mental Capacity Act was passed would still be valid. The Act sets out the criteria that must be met for an advance decision to be legally binding but this mainly echoes what was already the common law. Therefore, an existing advance decision may continue to be valid but it is advisable for the drafter – if he or she still retains capacity – to check that it meets the criteria in the Act. If it does not conform to the criteria and the patient already lacks capacity, much depends on other available evidence of the individual's wishes and legal advice may be needed. Even if not legally binding, a clear statement of the individual's wishes can be helpful in establishing what would be in that person's best interests and it should be taken into account.

While retaining capacity, patients are recommended to review their advance decisions periodically. Lack of review does not necessarily invalidate an advance decision but may raise questions about it. Obviously, when there are multiple copies of a document lodged with various relatives or health professionals, it is vital to ensure they are all up to date and patients must take steps to make clear if the decision has been retracted. Problems arise for health professionals if there is no indication of review, and treatment options or the individual's medical condition changed significantly prior to loss of capacity. Ideally, when they review their decision, people should indicate that they have done so. An updated document is more likely to be applicable to the circumstances. Outdated or badly drafted decisions cause confusion and can result in people not being treated as they had wished.

Storage of advance decisions

The main onus is on patients to make arrangements for any advance decision or advance care plan to be known about and for people close to the patient to be aware of its existence. Many people who make advance decisions give a copy to their GP. For chronically ill patients, who are treated by a specialist team over a prolonged period, a copy of the advance decision should be in both relevant hospital files and the GP record. Some people also carry a card, bracelet or other measure indicating the existence of an advance decision. As the National Programme for IT in the NHS develops, it may also be possible for patients to record the existence of their advance decision on the shared electronic record. Health professionals, once alerted to the existence of a relevant decision, should make reasonable efforts to find it. In an emergency, however, this may not be possible unless it is very promptly made available or registered on a system such as the electronic patient record.

Assessing whether an advance decision is legally binding

When time permits, efforts should be made to check the validity and applicability of any document presented. Basic verification includes checking that a written statement actually belongs to the patient who has been admitted, is dated, signed and witnessed. Emergency treatment should not be delayed in order to look for an advance decision if there is no clear indication that one exists. Nor should emergency measures be delayed if there are real doubts about the validity or applicability of an advance decision.

Health professionals need to consider whether:

- *the current circumstances match those envisaged in the advance decision;*
- *the decision is relevant to the patient's current health care needs;*
- *there is any evidence that the patient had a change of mind while retaining capacity;*
- *the decision, if old, has been reviewed (although this does not necessarily invalidate it);*
- *since the decision was last updated, new medical developments would have affected the patient's decision;*
- *the patient subsequently acted in a manner inconsistent with the decision made in the advance decision or subsequently appointed a proxy decision-maker to make the decision in question.*

The advance decision may not be binding if the current situation differs significantly from that which the patient anticipated. People who draft an advance decision knowing that they have a diagnosis likely to result eventually in loss of mental capacity may fail to envisage circumstances in the shorter term where an accident leaves them temporarily unconscious but capable of recovery. Anticipating the former, they may fail to make provision for the latter case, where they would want life-prolonging treatment provided. If an advance decision is not applicable to the circumstances, it is not legally binding although it may still give valuable indications of the general treatment options the patient would prefer. If a patient makes a statement that requests certain options, the health team will have to judge whether the treatment is medically appropriate or advisable for that patient at that time. If there is doubt about whether an advance decision is legally binding or not, a declaration should be sought from the Court of Protection in England and Wales, the High Court in Northern Ireland or the Court of Session in Scotland.

Conscientious objection

There is no clear legal right for health professionals to continue treating a patient because they have a conscientious objection to withdrawing life-prolonging treatment. They are entitled to their personal beliefs but cannot impose them on patients who do not share them and, in law, it may be an assault to continue treatment which the patient has refused. Arrangements may need to be made for health professionals without a conscientious objection to handle the patient's care. Clearly, transferring patients from one facility to another when they are seriously ill or near the end of life imposes hardship on them and their families but it may be the only option. In England and Wales, the Code of Practice of the Mental Capacity Act advises that if a transfer of care cannot be agreed voluntarily, the Court of Protection can direct those responsible for the care to make such arrangements. In an emergency, if no other health professional is available, health staff with a conscientious objection should not act contrary to a valid and applicable advance decision. It is ethically unacceptable and unlawful to force treatment upon a patient who has made a legally binding advance decision to refuse it.

Liability of health professionals

If an incapacitated patient is known to have objections to all or some treatment, health professionals need to consider the available evidence about the patient's views. In England and Wales, the Mental Capacity Act requires that the advance decision be in a written form if it refuses life-prolonging treatment. It must also meet the other criteria set out in the Act. In other parts of the United Kingdom, the common law position which is set out earlier in this chapter prevails. A valid and applicable written and witnessed treatment refusal is binding, unless retracted or unless a proxy was subsequently appointed to make the decision. Health care professionals are likely to be legally liable if they act contrary to it without good justification, such as evidence that its validity was suspect in some way. They are protected from liability if they:

- stop or do not initiate treatment that they reasonably believe has been refused by a valid and applicable advance decision;
- provide treatment if they have taken reasonable steps to find out if an advance decision exists but are unable to satisfy themselves that there is a valid and applicable advance decision.

Disputes and doubts about validity and applicability

In any case of doubt or dispute, legal judgment will be based upon the strength of the evidence about what the individual wanted. Where there is genuine doubt about the validity or applicability of an advance decision, there should be a presumption in favour of life and emergency treatment should be provided. Knowingly providing treatment in the face of a valid and applicable advance refusal, however, could result in legal action.

Initially, the clinician in charge of the incapacitated patient's care should consider the available evidence of the patient's former wishes and decide whether there is an advance decision which is valid and applicable to the circumstances. An advance request for positive interventions needs to be considered in the context of the individual's overall care and treatment options. There may be clinical reasons for not complying with a patient's requests, but if it is for life-prolonging treatment, attention needs to be given to the legal issues discussed earlier in relation to the Burke case.

Summary of chapter

- *Advance decision-making can be helpful for patients who know that they are likely to experience mental decline and have strong views about their future care. It can also relieve relatives of the burden of deciding and help health and care professionals assess the patient's best interests.*
- *Voluntariness is crucial and not everyone wants to plan in advance or have all the information they would need to do that in a valid and binding way.*
- *Informed refusals of treatment are binding if certain criteria are met but advance requests do not generally have the same legal force. It is important that patients are not given unrealistic expectations of what can be provided.*
- *Although advance refusals of life-prolonging treatment can have legal force, health professionals who have a conscientious objection to non-treatment should be able to opt out. They should make their views clear at an early stage of planning future care so that patients can make other arrangements.*

References

1. Help the Aged (2006). *Listening to Older People: Opening the Door for Older People to Explore End-of-Life Issues.* Help the Aged, London.
2. British Medical Association (2007). *Withholding and Withdrawing Life-Prolonging Medical Treatment: Guidance for Decision-Making: Third Edition.* BMA, London.
3. Re C (Adult: Refusal of Medical Treatment) [1994] 1 All ER 819.
4. See, for example, Airedale NHS Trust v Bland [1993] 1 All ER 821, Re T (Adult: Refusal of Treatment) [1992] 4 All ER 649.
5. R (on the application of Burke) v General Medical Council [2005] 2 FLR 1223 at 33.

Further resources

British Medical Association (2007). *Advance Decisions and Proxy Decisions in Medical Treatment and Research.* BMA, London.

British Medical Association, Resuscitation Council and Royal College of Nursing (2007). *Decisions Relating to Cardiopulmonary Resuscitation.* BMA, London.

Seymour J, Sanders C, Clarke A, et al. (2006). *Planning for Choice in End-of-Life Care.* Help the Aged, London.

Chapter 8 **Care at the end of life and preparing for a good death**

Living well and planning for end-of-life care

People are living longer and the disease patterns in their final years are changing. They may have chronic conditions such as cancer, cerebrovascular or respiratory diseases and other problems of varying severity, such as dementia, osteoporosis and arthritis. Most older people have more than one condition (multiple morbidity). Their care is likely to require co-ordination and collaboration among health and social care providers in different sectors and settings. Such liaison is essential for a good quality of life in older age when relatively minor problems can have significant psychological impact, especially if combined with physical or mental impairment, financial hardship and social isolation. The cumulative effect of several health problems can lead to greater impairment and higher care needs. In addition, older people are at greater risk of adverse drug reactions and complications resulting from treatment.

It is often difficult to predict the course of multiple chronic conditions, and care planning needs to be based on the holistic needs of each individual rather than on just a diagnosis. Personalised and dignified care which focuses on the individuality of each patient has been one of the themes running through the review of the NHS in 2007–8[1]. Also, in the United Kingdom, people have diverse cultural and religious beliefs which can make a significant difference to how they approach illness and death. Individual holistic assessment leading to appropriately tailored support is essential for living well in the final stages of life. Since the implementation of the National Service Framework for Older People, there has been an increased policy focus on positively maintaining the independence of older individuals. This is an important step towards promoting their quality of life. In addition, many older people want to acknowledge and plan for the certainty of death. When they want to discuss their fears and feelings about death, however, there may be few opportunities to do so.

The Ethics of Caring for Older People 2nd Edition. By British Medical Association. Published 2009 by Blackwell Publishing Limited, ISBN: 9781405176279.

Advance care planning (ACP)[2] is increasingly recognised as an essential process of discussion between individuals affected by a life-limiting condition, their families and their care providers of various disciplines. It provides a framework within which people can talk about their values, goals, their understanding of their prognosis and preferences for care. It differs from general care planning because it takes place in the context of an anticipated deterioration in the individual's condition, with a possible attendant loss of mental capacity. Many people appreciate the chance to prepare themselves and their families for the inevitable, but as with any form of care planning, it should not be forced on people who are reluctant to think about the likelihood of deteriorating physical or mental health.

Provision of information and discussing death

Explicit ACP can be reassuring for many older people, and professionals providing palliative care are accustomed to engaging in such activity. Other health and social care providers, however, are sometimes reluctant to discuss end-of-life care, fearing that the message will be interpreted as the end of hope. In a culture which often emphasises cure rather than care, acknowledging the inevitability of death can seem like accepting failure. Even when there is no chance of improvement, patients often want information to help them prepare. Details need to be both truthfully and sensitively explained, so that people do not have unrealistic expectations about what is achievable, in terms of predicting or controlling the dying process. It is not always possible to foretell when and how death will occur. Empathy and moral support are important, but allowing unrealistic expectations to develop is unfair for everyone, including the health and social care professionals.

Individuals' reluctance or readiness to acknowledge their own illness and death is a key factor in any discussion. An overemphasis on completing advance care plans can give the impression that this is something they must do. Involving everyone in planning for approaching death is inappropriate because some people refuse to contemplate it. However, the amount of information that older people want is frequently underestimated. Most people want to know their diagnosis but there is more diversity of views about the amount of information they want about the progression of the disease[3]. When the charity, Help the Aged, asked older people's feelings about discussing the end of life, many responded saying things like 'we prepare for everything except the one thing that comes to us all'. Some particularly regretted that death in care homes happens behind closed doors, rather than allowing or encouraging friends to sit with the dying person and talk about their fears[4]. A project examining people's feelings as they near the end of life showed that they sometimes felt frustrated and isolated because of the unwillingness of family and carers to discuss their death[5]. One participant exclaimed, 'But no one asks me how I feel. I find it really upsetting the way they desperately avoid the subject … Don't they get it? I'm going to die!' Another participant reported how seeing a female patient on the ward, after she had died, helped allay fears of her own imminent death. Not everyone would want this, just as not everyone feels ready to discuss their illness or approaching death but there should be opportunities for discussion for those who do.

Discussion of death is not customary in some other cultures but assumptions should not be made solely on the basis of a person's culture or ethnicity. Chinese older people who participated in the series of 'listening events' undertaken by Help the Aged[6] said that, in their culture, it was bad luck to talk about death but they personally welcomed the chance of frank discussion. The World Health Organization (WHO) has highlighted how older cancer patients generally 'want more information, want to be involved in decision-making and experience better psychological adjustment if palliative care and good communication are part of their care from the time of diagnosis'[7]. Despite some relatives' requests that information be withheld from older cancer sufferers, 88% of patients aged from 65 to 94 years wanted to know more[8]. Other conditions such as heart disease appear to stimulate less open communication and, in this respect, the management of such conditions compares unfavourably in terms of information and support, with that available to cancer patients[8]. People need to know what to expect in the period leading up to their death. For many, loss of control is one of their main fears and having the opportunity to plan can have a positive psychological effect. They may also need to take practical steps to put their affairs in order, ensure a will is up-to-date, sort out finances or seek reconciliation with relatives. Open discussion and ACP can help to achieve this and ensure that all involved in the individual's care are aware of that person's problems and wishes.

Help the Aged found that, compared to younger terminally ill patients, older people have fewer opportunities to discuss treatment options or other problems they experience. They are:

- *less likely to die in the place they would prefer to;*
- *less likely to receive specialist care;*
- *more likely to have multiple health problems;*
- *less likely to have social support networks;*
- *more likely to have financial difficulties.*

Honesty and truth telling

Good communication is discussed in Chapter 2 where honesty between health professionals and patients, as well as clear communication between care providers, is emphasised. Professionals' ability to recognise the key signs of people approaching their last days is important for planning a good end of life, even though death is not always predictable. At this stage, members of the care team need to communicate particularly well with each other, with the individual and the family. It is important to avoid mixed messages which lead to poor management. Once dying is diagnosed, care needs to refocus. Relatives and older people themselves may initially collude with a pretence that death is not approaching but then feel aggrieved and unprepared when the truth emerges. It is better for health and social care professionals sensitively to explore patients' wishes, with the aim of encouraging them to recognise the reality of their situation. A frequent source of anger and dismay among bereaved relatives is that they were not specifically told that their relative was dying. Most people want their families involved in decisions but if they do not want relatives informed of the prognosis, confidentiality should be maintained. That is not to say that older people cannot be encouraged, if willing, to consider the desirability of preparing their relatives. Vital last opportunities for closeness and reconciliation may otherwise be lost. Part of the general perception of a 'good death' involves patients and those close to them supporting each other.

Palliative care

The guidelines on palliative care published by the National Institute for Clinical Excellence (NICE) emphasise the need for support at all stages of a person's experience of life-threatening illness. They define 'palliative care' as the alleviation of pain and discomfort to improve a person's quality of life when a cure is not possible[9]. When people reach the terminal stages of illness, the palliative model, which was originally developed in hospices, focuses on bringing together physical, psychological, social, emotional and spiritual facets of care. Clinically, the focus at this point is on keeping the person comfortable and free from distressing symptoms, but palliative care can also be helpful in the earlier stages of illness alongside other therapies which are intended to prolong life. Although opinions differ as to what a good death involves, most agree it is one in which pain and distress are well managed, the dying person and his or her relatives feel supported rather than abandoned and a sense of closure is achieved. Helping people to prepare for their own death, and their relatives to prepare for bereavement, requires a range of skills. Evidence-based guidelines are available on facets such as symptom control, psychosocial support and bereavement care (see 'Further resources' at the end of the chapter).

When people enter the 'dying stage' of illness, their treatment needs to be reassessed. Several tools exist to assist this process and ensure that care is provided in as coherent a manner as possible. In primary care, the Gold Standards Framework[10] aims to develop a locally based system to improve the organisation and quality of care for people in the last year of life. It can improve communication and co-ordination so that more people who wish to die at home can do so. The Preferred Priorities for Care questionnaire[11] helps individuals formulate their own lists of preferences and priorities and provides a way for them to discuss these with family and friends. Perhaps the best-known tool, however, is the Liverpool Care Pathway for the Dying Patient (LCP) which is a model of best practice for care in the last few days of life and is implemented across the United Kingdom. This multidisciplinary document replaces the medical and nursing notes and aims to reduce the amount of paperwork to focus on symptom management and the need to only document changes around this. It was developed in order to transfer the hospice model of end-of-life care into other settings, including hospitals and care homes, and to enable health and social care professionals to deliver a model of excellence in end-of-life care. Although the model was originally developed for cancer sufferers, it has been adapted to the management of patients with other diseases.

The LCP is implemented after the health care team has agreed that the person has entered the dying phase and provides a holistic model of care for both patients and their relatives before and after the individual's death. The pathway sets out a series of goals to be addressed, which include discontinuing inappropriate treatment, ensuring the individual's spiritual needs are addressed and checking that communication with family members is effective. The main goals of the LCP are summarised below and further information about it is available in 'Further resources' at the end of this chapter.

Goals in care for dying patients (adapted from the LCP)

Comfort measures
- *Medication assessed and non-essentials discontinued.*
- *Subcutaneous drugs as appropriate for pain, agitation, nausea, etc.*
- *Discontinue inappropriate interventions which may include intravenous fluids.*
- *Document not for CPR.*

Psychological and insight issues
- *Ability to communicate assessed and translator obtained if required.*

> * *Individual's insight into condition assessed.*
> *Religious and spiritual support*
> * *Religious and spiritual needs assessed with patient and family.*
> *Communication with family or others*
> * *Identify which people need to be informed of the impending death and how.*
> *Communication with primary health care providers*
> * *GP informed.*
> *Summary*
> * *Care plan discussed with patient and family.*

Disadvantaged groups – advocacy and listening to patients

The palliative care model provides a standard of excellence for terminal care but older people are described as the 'disadvantaged dying'[12] because they are less likely to receive palliative care. Resource issues partly account for this as, although about 24% of people would like to die in a hospice, there are hospice beds only for about 4%[13]. Older people from black and ethnic minorities have even lower access to palliative care services and the reasons for this are unclear. Among possible explanations are a lack of awareness among those communities of the potential benefits and the perception, among older people and professionals alike, that palliative care is for cancer rather than for conditions which are more prevalent among people from black and ethnic minority backgrounds, such as heart disease and strokes. It is true that palliative care historically grew from caring for cancer patients, who remain the main recipients of specialist palliative care services. As cancer has generally been a less prevalent killer disease amongst some first and second generation immigrant groups, this may also contribute to their lower rate of access to palliative care. The disparities may also be attributable to general social and material deprivation rather than ethnicity. The Policy Research Institute on Ageing and Ethnicity (PRIAE) has identified some reasons to account for the lack of uptake among some groups. One is the stereotype that underlies some social policy and planning that ethnic and minority extended families tend to 'look after their own' so that specific service provision for them is less essential. Individuals themselves also often lack accessible information about services and advocacy[14]. The PRIAE report saw poor 'information and communication which suggests that there is an information gap in service provision'. It recommended more information in minority languages and better liaison with voluntary organisations in black and ethnic minority communities. Cultural differences were also seen as contributory to the lack of access to services by such groups. Patients from African, Caribbean, south Asian and Chinese communities are sometimes unfamiliar with complex UK service structures. Health and social care staff are also often unfamiliar with clients' and patients' cultural values. (This is also flagged up in Chapters 1 and 2.)

Case example – the need to avoid stereotyping

B was a lady of 70 who came to the United Kingdom as an asylum seeker with her granddaughter who was her sole relative. Both were given leave to remain due to their legitimate fear of persecution in their country of origin. Other members of B's family, including her son to whom she had been close, had died in ethnic violence. B had some knowledge of English but she tended to become very agitated when questioned and usually her granddaughter translated for her. B was seen as a difficult and demanding person, sometimes described as 'attention-seeking' or 'histrionic' in her repeated visits to her GP. Although B appeared to have various health problems, including what she claimed were bouts of acute pain, the consensus was that her core problems were psychological. Her various ailments were thought to stem from distress and trauma from becoming a refugee late in life. It was thought that she was suffering from post-traumatic stress disorder. B was prescribed anti-depressants but it was only after 18 months that she was eventually diagnosed as having cancer which had been previously missed. B had been frustrated and distressed by her inability to communicate in English but it also seemed that those treating her had failed to listen attentively enough and some false assumptions had been made about her condition, based on negative stereotyping.

Arranging religious and spiritual care for those who wish it

End-of-life care must be sensitive to individuals' personal, cultural and spiritual values. The NICE guidelines[9] on palliative care identify the need to meet a person's spiritual needs as one of the four domains of palliative care. For many, the spiritual dimension is immensely important. This is not restricted to people who have a religious belief. People who are not religious often also want to have support to help them think about the values that have been important to them throughout life as they come to terms with death. Humanist advisers can sometimes fulfil this role, as well as hospital chaplains, rabbis, imams or other faith-based spiritual advisers. In a multi-faith, multi-cultural society such as the United Kingdom, it is important that professionals providing care and support to people nearing the end of life take account of individuals' varying spiritual needs. Ideally, these should be assessed before people reach the terminal or dying phase of illness. This gives them time to explore issues that may be troubling them before they reach the very end of life[15]. The people involved in the Help the Aged listening events mentioned earlier felt that health care professionals generally and nurses in particular could usefully be more alert to patients' spiritual needs[4]. Some people wish to observe specific traditions at the end of life or in the care of the body after death. The LCP emphasises the importance of identifying and respecting cultural and religious customs before and after death.

Last weeks and the place of death

When people talk about where they would like to die, what they usually mean is they would like to choose where they will be cared for in the period immediately preceding their death, not just where death should take place. Most older people die in hospital but this is not usually their preference. Some would prefer to spend their last weeks in a hospice or specialist palliative care unit, either because they feel safer there or in order to relieve their family of the responsibility and burdens of care. Many want to remain at home for as long as possible and only be transferred to a specialist in-patient unit when death approaches. Although people's preferences about the place of death should be accommodated where possible, this is not always practical if relatives cannot provide home care or sufficient professional support cannot be put in place. The commonest reasons for admission to hospital or a hospice are breakdown of carer arrangements and problems controlling the patient's symptoms. Around a fifth of deaths of people over the age of 65 occur in care homes, but there is a trend of older patients being moved from care homes to hospital just before death[16]. Wherever possible, this should be avoided so that older people do not undergo unplanned transfers in the last days or hours of life. In the past, there was a lack of palliative care in residential settings but it should be available for everyone needing it. Nowadays, many Community Palliative Care teams visit residential nursing homes. Medical support is essential, including out-of-hours care and good interagency co-operation. In care home or domestic settings palliative care should ideally be provided by the individual's usual professional carers, although access to specialist services may also be needed. For care home residents, this is their actual home and they should receive the same access to NHS services that they would have had in their former dwelling.

Team and inter-agency co-operation

Although ultimately the responsibility for deciding what treatment to offer rests with the clinician in charge of the patient's care, it is important, where non-emergency decisions are made, that account is taken of the views of other professionals involved. Good communication and team-working is particularly important in an individual's care at the end of life. Professionals, including care assistants, who have insight into the older person's wishes or have spent a lot of time with the patient and relatives can make a particularly valuable contribution. When older people lack capacity, as well as their GP who might be able to throw light on their former wishes, any appointed proxy needs to be involved. Chapter 4 discusses proxy decision-makers with lasting power of attorney under the Mental Capacity Act in England and Wales, and welfare attorneys and guardians appointed under the Adults with Incapacity Act in Scotland.

Fairness and avoidance of discrimination

Health professionals must ensure that treatment decisions are based on a proper assessment of the relevant factors in each individual case, rather than on assumptions about the person's age, appearance, behaviour or disability. Decisions to withhold or withdraw life-sustaining treatment are more common among older people who are more likely to have multiple morbidity. Their clinical condition may make some interventions too risky but this may give the appearance of unfair discrimination against them. It is important that the reasons for not offering some life-sustaining treatments are clearly communicated to patients who have capacity or to those representing patients who lack capacity. Such decisions should also be clearly articulated and recorded in the notes.

Whether to provide or withhold conventional treatments – older people with capacity

Few issues in medicine are more complex and difficult than those addressed by older people, their relatives and health professionals concerning the decision to withhold or withdraw potentially life-sustaining measures. Treatments such as renal dialysis can prolong life but cannot reverse a patient's disease or underlying condition. For people of any age, some treatments which might provide a therapeutic benefit are not inevitably given but are weighed according to a number of factors, such as the individual's wishes, the treatment's invasiveness and likely success, side effects, limits of efficacy and the resources available. When a particular treatment cannot provide a sustainable benefit, the main reason for offering it no longer

exists. Most treatments entail some risks as well as benefits, and the justification for giving a treatment disappears if the net benefit does not outweigh the harms and risks. As is also discussed in Chapters 4 and 7, health
professionals are legally bound by an individual's valid (advance or contemporaneous) refusal of treatment. Decisions by health professionals to
discontinue a treatment, which is judged to no longer provide any benefit
when the recipient is willing to continue it, need very sensitive discussion
with that person. It is important that all those involved in the decision –
including the individual – understand the reasons for the decision, the
grounds on which it needs to be made and the implications. Health professionals have an obligation to ensure that reliable data are used to make
such decisions, rather than rely on assumptions about people's wishes or
assumptions about their ability to gain benefit, even at an advanced age.
Such decisions for people with impaired capacity are discussed below.

'Essential nursing care'

Some types of care should never be withheld. These are sometimes referred
to as 'basic care' or, more properly, 'essential nursing care'. The term speaks
for itself and is generally accepted to cover those interventions which keep
individuals in a dignified, clean and comfortable situation. It includes offering them food, liquids, pain relief, hygiene measures and management of
distressing symptoms, such as breathlessness and vomiting. Near the end of
life, people seldom want nutrition or hydration but essential nursing care
includes measures such as moistening an individual's mouth for comfort.
Whilst some medical treatments may be withheld, appropriate comfort care
should always be provided unless actively resisted by the person. This does
not mean that all facets of care must be provided in all cases. When mentally competent people refuse pain relief, for example, because they want
to remain alert and able to interact with those around them, their decision
should be respected, although analgesics should continue to be offered. When
the individual is unable to express preferences, procedures that are essential
to keep that person comfortable should always be offered and this should
be discussed with any appointed proxy decision-maker (see Chapter 4).
The presumption should be in favour of providing relief from symptoms
and distress and enhancing the older person's dignity.

Whether to provide or withhold conventional treatments – older people with impaired capacity

Under the Mental Capacity Act in England and Wales and the common law
in Northern Ireland, decisions made on behalf of people who lack mental

capacity must be made in their 'best interests'. In Scotland, decisions are made on the basis of what would 'benefit' the incapacitated individual. (Best interests and benefit are similar concepts and are discussed in Chapters 3 and 4.) Frequently, it benefits people and is in their best interests to receive life-sustaining treatment. This is true of patients at any age, but care providers need to take particular care to ensure that decisions for older people are made fairly and without discrimination. The legal criteria which must be taken into account in assessing any incapacitated person's best interests are set out in Chapter 4, which also discusses how a range of proxy decision-makers should be involved in decisions affecting incapacitated adults. Close relatives of the patient, welfare attorneys, deputies or Independent Mental Capacity Advocates may need to be consulted, depending on the prior arrangements made for protecting the individual's best interests. The respective codes of practice for the Mental Capacity Act and the Adults with Incapacity (Scotland) Act provide further guidance[17]. The issues discussed in Chapter 7 regarding people's advance wishes about end-of-life care are also relevant here as part of the assessment of what would be in their best interests or would benefit them. The type of factors that need to be considered when specifically considering withdrawing or withholding life-sustaining treatment include:

• the person's known wishes, including any written statements made when the person had capacity;
• clinical judgement about the effectiveness of the proposed treatment;
• the likelihood of the person experiencing severe unmanageable pain or suffering;
• the level of awareness individuals have of their existence and surroundings;
• the likelihood and extent of any degree of improvement if treatment is provided;
• whether the invasiveness, risks and side effects of the treatment are justified in the circumstances;
• the views of any appointed health care proxy or welfare attorney (see Chapter 4);
• the views of people close to the person, especially close relatives, partners and carers, about what the individual is likely to see as beneficial.

In the case of Mr Burke (discussed in Chapter 7), the Appeal Court considering the general issue of when life-sustaining treatment might not be in a person's interests said that where 'life involves an extreme degree of pain, discomfort or indignity to a patient, who is sentient but not competent and who has manifested no wish to be kept alive', the courts accept that it may not be in that person's interests to be kept alive artificially[18].

When, after appropriate consultation with those close to the incapacitated individual, a decision is made to withhold or withdraw a particular treatment, the reasons for this should be carefully explained so that it is not interpreted by relatives as 'giving up on' or abandoning the patient. They need to understand that life-sustaining treatment should be withdrawn if it cannot benefit the individual or if that person has previously refused it by an advance decision. The aim is to ensure that treatment which is no longer in the best interests of the person is avoided[19]. It is only lawful to withhold or withdraw treatment when to continue it is not in the incapacitated person's best interests. The courts have confirmed that, in such circumstances, the health team would not be in breach of its duty to protect life under the Human Rights Act[20].

Case example – withholding treatment

J suffered a stroke after which he never recovered his mental capacity. He remained incontinent and severely physically disabled but was able to accept food and drink. He was discharged home into the care of his son and daughter-in-law who, with a lot of support from the community health care team and the GP, provided a high standard of care for J. He had been a keen gardener before his stroke and seemed particularly to enjoy being wheeled into the garden. After several months, however, J had to be readmitted to hospital with a respiratory infection. He recovered after antibiotic treatment and appeared to continue to enjoy aspects of his life despite his incapacity and physical disability. Soon after, he developed a more serious respiratory tract infection, became critically ill and was placed on a ventilator. The family and health team discussed whether it would be appropriate to carry out a tracheotomy but it was felt that J was too ill to survive it and that continuing with ventilation was also inappropriate as it could not restore him to a situation where he could leave hospital. After further discussion, J's treatment was withdrawn, with his family's agreement.

Oral nutrition and hydration

Where nutrition and hydration are provided by ordinary means – such as by cup, spoon or any other method for delivering food or nutritional supplements into a person's mouth – or the moistening of the mouth for comfort, this normally forms part of essential nursing care. Competent people can refuse food and water but these fundamental facets of care should always be offered. Usually, it would be a benefit or in the best interests of incapacitated people to have food and drink by these means, unless that would cause choking or aspiration of food or fluid. They should not, however, be forced to eat and drink if they resist. Where oral feeding is unable to meet the nutritional needs of the individual, formal consideration should be given to providing ANH (see the next section). It is also important that older people who need help to eat and drink are assisted. Failure to provide them with adequate nutrition and hydration, or failure to provide assistance to those who need it, constitute neglect on the part of care providers. As is discussed in Chapter 2, it may also be elder abuse. While nutrition and hydration should not be forced upon patients who express a clear refusal, it is important to find out why they are reluctant to eat and whether, for example, they have a religious objection to the particular food offered. Many older people with a disability require assistance with feeding but retain the ability to swallow if the food is placed in their mouth; this forms part of essential nursing care. When people are close to death, they seldom want nutrition and/or hydration and its provision may, in fact, exacerbate their discomfort. Good practice must, however, include good oral care to avoid the discomfort of a dry mouth.

Artificial nutrition and hydration

Provision or non-provision of ANH can be a controversial area where views differ. Some people regard artificial feeding as basic or essential care which should be provided unless the person is dying. Judgements in legal cases in England and Scotland[21], however, have classified ANH as medical treatments which – like any other medical intervention – may not be provided or can be withdrawn in some circumstances. Competent people can refuse such interventions and they can only be provided when in the best interests of incapacitated people. It is established in common law that decisions not to insert a feeding tube, or not to reinsert it if it becomes dislodged, are medical decisions. They are taken after assessment of the individual circumstances of the case. As discussed earlier, a decision to stop providing ordinary nutrition and hydration, however, is not a medical treatment in the same way but part of essential nursing care.

When people of any age are in the terminal stage of life, it is not usually appropriate to provide such invasive treatment as ANH but the individual circumstances must always be considered. In cases where people are not terminally ill and near death, safeguards must be in place to ensure that appropriate consideration is given to their individual circumstances. The General Medical Council's (GMC) guidance, which is binding on all doctors, requires that a second clinical opinion is sought before ANH is withheld or withdrawn from a person who is not imminently dying. This opinion should be sought from a senior clinician (medical or nursing) who has experience of the person's condition and who is not directly involved in the individual's care[22]. This is to ensure that, in this most sensitive area, the person's interests have been thoroughly considered and to provide reassurance to those close to patients and the wider public.

Although ANH are often classed together, there are good clinical reasons why hydration and nutrition should be assessed separately. For example, with some terminally ill patients, subcutaneous or intravenous fluids may avoid dehydration, decrease pressure sore risk and aid comfort, but the provision of nutrition artificially would be too invasive to be in a person's best interests. With other people, it is appropriate for both nutrition and hydration to be provided, withheld or withdrawn.

The law relating to withdrawal of ANH can be complex, as is shown by the case of Burke v GMC, discussed in Chapter 7. If a person is assessed as being in a persistent vegetative state (PVS) or in a state of very low awareness closely resembling PVS, and not imminently dying, any proposal to withdraw ANH requires legal review in England, Wales and Northern Ireland. In Scotland, the withdrawal of ANH from a person in PVS does not require a court declaration in the same way. Further advice on this is provided in the British Medical Association's book *Withholding and Withdrawing Life-Prolonging Medical Treatment: Guidance for Decision-Making* (see 'Further resources' at the end of the chapter).

Disagreements about treatment withdrawal

In most cases, after the issues have been discussed, agreement is reached between the health care team, the individual, or individual's family or the proxy decision-maker about the best way to proceed. When disagreement arises, steps should be taken to address the issue without delay. Further information, discussion and seeking a second opinion can resolve some difficulties, but where these fail, legal advice should be sought. Many disagreements can be resolved without the need for a full court hearing. Sometimes lawyers are able to give advice about how to proceed or a judge may make the decision in a medical emergency. It is important to remember that the law can provide a protective role for both patients and the health care team who treat them and where there is disagreement that cannot be quickly resolved, legal advice should be sought. Health professionals should not be deterred from seeking a legal ruling because of the risk of appearing confrontational. If the situation cannot be resolved through discussion and good communication, legal review can be beneficial for all parties.

Case example – flawed team working

A GP was providing care for his 85-year-old patient, Mrs X, in a nursing home. Mrs X had suffered a series of strokes and was unable to swallow. She was fed by food supplements being placed into her mouth by syringe. In June 1995, the doctor gave instructions to the nursing staff that the food supplements should be stopped. The nursing staff disagreed with these instructions and continued to feed Mrs X secretly until the supplements ran out. Mrs X died in late August 1995. The doctor was reported to the GMC, which found him guilty of serious professional misconduct for failing to follow proper procedures in reaching the decision to withdraw the food supplements. In particular, it was found that he had failed to seek a second opinion when he should have done and failed adequately to seek or heed the views of the nursing staff[23].

Cardiopulmonary resuscitation

CPR attempts to restore breathing and spontaneous circulation in patients who have suffered cardiac and/or respiratory arrest. It can be very invasive, including chest compression, electric shock, injection of drugs and ventilation although electric shock alone can sometimes restore cardiac function. Patients and their families are often unaware of what is involved or that survival rates after cardiorespiratory arrest and CPR are extremely low. They may also be unaware that attempting resuscitation carries risks, such as rib or sternal fractures, hepatic or splenic rupture or that patients may be left with brain damage. It cannot prolong the life of people who are imminently dying from an injury or disease process but it can make their death more unpleasant. Patients for whom it is likely to be an option (or their relatives if patients themselves are mentally incapacitated) need to know what is involved. People who have cared for relatives who underwent attempted CPR are far more aware of these risks and often less willing to accept them for themselves. In the discussions organised by Help the Aged, for example, some older people who had cared for relatives in that situation decided that they would not want CPR to be attempted on themselves. The British Medical Association and Royal College of Nursing and Resuscitation Council (United Kingdom) have jointly issued detailed guidance on CPR decisions (see 'Further resources' at the end of this chapter).

When to discuss CPR

Chapter 7 deals with advance decision-making and also the issue of do-not-attempt-resuscitation (DNAR) decisions which are made in advance. If no

DNAR decision has previously been made, health professionals are sometimes unclear about when, and in what situations, they should talk to older people about CPR and when it would be inappropriate to raise the subject. If older people themselves or their relatives raise questions about CPR, or want to discuss whether it would be likely to work for them, they should be answered truthfully and the facts discussed. As with individuals of all ages, where older people have existing conditions which make cardiac arrest likely, consideration should be given in advance to formulating a management plan. In some cases, earlier general discussions with older people will have already established such a care and treatment plan, including mention of palliative care and CPR. The LCP, for example, prompts clinicians to consider and document the patient's CPR status at the initial assessment stage. Health care professionals can help people, who are willing to do so, to plan for their future care in a sensitive and realistic manner, and this can include making it clear whether or not attempted CPR is likely to be needed and successful. In some cases, the clinical issues are straightforward. If, after looking at the person's medical history, the health care team concludes that CPR would be very unlikely to be successful in restarting the heart and maintaining respiration in that person's case if cardiac arrest occurred, it should not be offered. An extreme example would be a patient in the final stages of a terminal illness for whom death is approaching. CPR is unlikely to work and could increase the individual's suffering.

Decisions about attempting CPR raise very sensitive and potentially distressing issues for patients and people emotionally close to them. Some health professionals find it difficult to discuss the subject with patients but need to do so if cardiac arrest is likely to occur and CPR could be successful, but it is unclear how the person feels about the risks involved. In advance discussion of cases where CPR is likely to restart the patient's heart for a sustained period, the benefits and risks should be discussed with competent individ-uals and with those close to patients who lack capacity. Any such decisions, and the reasons for them, should be recorded in the medical notes.

It is not necessary to raise the issue if it is clear that CPR would not be successful, if the person has already refused it or if the patient has reached the terminal stage of life. Dying patients should not be subjected to CPR as this would be futile and inappropriate. Occasionally, individuals or their relatives request that CPR be attempted in situations where the health care team consider it futile and clinically inappropriate. Where the clinical view is that CPR would not restart the heart and breathing, this needs to be explained in a sensitive way. Health professionals should not agree to provide treatment which is clinically inappropriate but such discussions with patients are obviously very difficult and should be led by an experienced clinician, where possible.

When to attempt CPR

As mentioned earlier, for some patients, such as those in the final stages of a terminal illness for whom death is imminent, CPR is inappropriate. For other people, where there is no DNAR order in place, no proper assessment has been made and the person's wishes are unknown; the presumption is that all reasonable efforts are made to revive him or her. Sometimes when CPR is started in such an emergency situation, clinical information soon emerges indicating that it is very unlikely to succeed and it would be inappropriate to continue.

CPR should never be attempted on people who have refused it but assumptions should not be made about older people's wishes if the issue has not been discussed with them. It is sometimes erroneously assumed that older people who have multiple morbidity and a relatively poor prognosis should not be considered for CPR. In fact, it is important that advance consideration be given to the issue and decisions made on a case-by-case basis. Blanket decisions against CPR solely on the basis of age or disability, rather than the individual's actual condition, could raise questions of unfair discrimination. In some cases, however, it may not be a question of providing the full panoply of CPR technology but ensuring that personnel are trained to provide basic CPR. All establishments that face decisions about attempting CPR including hospitals, general practices, care homes and ambulance services, should have a clear policy about it. These policies must be readily available to and understood by staff[24].

Case example – attempting CPR despite a DNAR decision

N was a 76-year-old patient with a heart condition which made it unlikely that CPR would be able to restart her heart and keep it functioning in the event of a serious heart attack or stroke. She was aware of this and, as part of a her long-term care plan, a DNAR decision had been placed in her medical record. In other respects, she was in reasonably good health and enjoyed her life. She went into hospital for a minor procedure on her foot, involving regional anaesthesia. Unfortunately, this triggered an unexpected cardio-respiratory instability. Her medical notes said not for resuscitation but the DNAR decision had not been intended to cover an easily reversible cause of potential cardiorespiratory arrest. The clinician in charge of N's care decided that resuscitation must be immediately started and the DNAR decision suspended as it had not been intended to apply to the situation which developed. In this instance, it was successful and N enjoyed several further years of life.

In some exceptional cases such as the example mentioned earlier, patients with whom a DNAR decision has been agreed may experience cardiac or respiratory arrest from a reversible cause such as choking, induction of anaesthesia or a severe allergic reaction. In those kinds of cases where the condition can be successfully reversed, resuscitation is appropriate, unless the patient has previously specifically refused it with that kind of situation in mind.

Summary of advice on CPR

- *Decisions about CPR must be made on the basis of an individual assessment of each person's case.*
- *ACP is an important part of good care for those at risk of cardiorespiratory arrest.*
- *Communication and the provision of information are essential parts of good quality care.*
- *It is not necessary to initiate discussion about CPR with individuals if there is no reason to believe that they are likely to suffer a cardiorespiratory arrest.*
- *Generally where no explicit decision has been made in advance, there should be an initial presumption in favour of CPR, but if CPR would not restart the heart and breathing, it should not be attempted.*
- *Where the expected benefit of attempted CPR is outweighed by the burdens, the person's own views are important.*
- *If the individual lacks capacity, an appointed proxy decision-maker or those close to that person should be involved in discussions.*
- *If a person with capacity refuses CPR, or a person lacking capacity has a valid and applicable advance decision refusing CPR, this should be respected.*
- *A DNAR decision does not override clinical judgement should the cause of the patient's respiratory or cardiac arrest be reversible and not match the circumstances envisaged.*
- *DNAR decisions apply only to CPR and not to any other aspects of treatment.*

Summary of chapter

- *Good communication between different care providers is particularly important in the care of older people as they are more likely than younger patients to suffer from multiple conditions.*
- *For many people, loss of control is one of their main fears. Individuals should have opportunities to discuss this, their illness, prognosis and fears about death but should not be pushed to do so, if they are unwilling.*

- Care should be individually tailored and encompass physical, psychological, social and spiritual aspects of care. In so far as possible, individual preferences of place of death should be met.
- Honesty and truth-telling are crucial facets of good communication at the end of life. Poor communication and lack of clear information are frequent sources of anger for bereaved relatives.
- Difficult decisions to withhold or withdraw life-prolonging treatment arise if that treatment would not or can no longer provide sustained benefit to the patient. Reasons for not providing life-prolonging treatment must be clearly communicated to individuals who have capacity or those close to people who lack capacity.
- CPR status should be considered for all individuals whose condition makes cardiac arrest likely.
- CPR is not appropriate when patients reach the dying stage of their illness.

References

1. Department of Health (2007). Our NHS Our Future: NHS Next Stage Review, Interim Report (2008) High Quality Care for All: NHS Next Stage Review Final Report. DH, London.
2. NHS End of Life Care Progamme (2007). *Advance Care Planning: A Guide for Health and Social Care Staff.* DH, London.
3. See, for example, Meredith C, Symonds P, Webster L, et al. (1996). Information needs of cancer patients in West Scotland: cross sectional survey of patients' views. *Br Med J* **313**: 724–6.
4. Help the Aged (2006). *Listening to Older People: Opening the Door for Older People to Explore End-of-Life Issues.* Help the Aged, London.
5. Schels W, Moorhead J. (2008). Life before death. Wellcome Collection Exhibition 9 April 2008–18 May 2008. *The Guardian* 1/4/2008.
6. Seymour J, Sanders C, Clarke A, et al. (2006). *Planning for Choice in End-of-Life Care.* Help the Aged, London.
7. World Health Organization Europe. Davies E, Higginson IJ (eds) (2004). *Better Palliative Care for Older People.* WHO, Copenhagen, p. 16.
8. Ajaj A, Singh MP, Abdulla AJJ (2001). Should elderly patients be told they have cancer? Questionnaire survey of older people. *Br Med J* **323**: 1160.
9. National Institute for Clinical Excellence (2004). Supportive and palliative care services for adults with cancer. NICE, London.
10. The Gold Standards Framework (GSF): a programme for community palliative care. The GSF was incorporated into the NHS End of Life Care Programme in April 2005.
11. Preferred Priorities for Care (2007) originated by Lancashire & South Cumbria Cancer Network and endorsed by the NHS End of Life Care Programme.
12. Harris L (1990). Continuing care: the disadvantaged dying. *Nursing Times* **86**(22): 26–9.

13. National Council for Palliative Care (2006). *End of Life Care Strategy. The National Council of Palliative Care Submission.* NCPC, London.
14. The Policy Research Institute on Ageing and Ethnicity (2000). *Black and Minority Ethnic Elders in the UK: Health & Social Care Research Findings.* PRIAE, Leeds.
15. Speck P (2003). Spiritual/religious issues in care of the dying. In: Ellershaw J, Wilkinson S (eds) *Care of the Dying. A Pathway to Excellence.* University of Oxford Press, Oxford, pp. 90–105.
16. Help the Aged (2005). *Dying in Older Age: Reflections from an Older Person's Perspective.* Help the Aged, London.
17. Mental Capacity Act Code of Practice, Adults with Incapacity (Scotland) Act Code of Practice. The Scottish Government, Edinburgh.
18. R (on the application of Burke) v General Medical Council [2005] 2 FLR 1223 at 33.
19. R v Woollin [1998] 4 All ER 103.
20. NHS Trust A v M; NHS Trust B v H [2001] 1 All ER 801.
21. See, for example, Frenchay Healthcare NHS Trust v S [1994] 1 WLR 601, Re D (Medical Treatment) [1998] 1 FLR 411 and Law Hospital NHS Trust v Lord Advocate (1996) SLT 848.
22. General Medical Council (2002). *Withholding and Withdrawing Life-Prolonging Treatments: Good Practice in Decision-Making.* GMC, London. At the time of writing, this GMC guidance is being revised.
23. General Medical Council Professional Conduct Committee hearing, 15–16 and 18–26 March 1999.
24. NHS Executive (2000). Resuscitation policy (HSC 2000/028). Department of Health, London. Scottish Executive Health Department (2000). Resuscitation policy (HDL [2000] 22). Scottish Executive, Edinburgh.

Further resources

British Medical Association (2007). *Withholding and Withdrawing Life-Prolonging Medical Treatment: Third Edition.* Blackwell Publishing, London. The National Council for Palliative Care has also published guidance (2007) *Artificial Nutrition and Hydration – Guidance in End of Life Care for Adults.*

Liverpool Care Pathway. Ellershaw J, Wilkinson S (2003). *Care of the Dying: A Pathway to Excellence.* Oxford University Press, Oxford.

National Council for Palliative Care Services (2006). *Changing Gear: Guidelines for Managing the Last Days of Life: The Research Evidence.* NCPC, London.

Neuberger J (1987). *Caring for Dying People of Different Faiths.* Lisa Sainsbury Foundation, London.

The National Council for Palliative Care and the NHS End of Life Care Programme (2007). *Building on Firm Foundations. Improving End-of-Life Care in Care Homes: Examples of Innovative Practice.* NCPC, London.

The National Gold Standards Framework: Programme for Community Palliative Care. NGSF, Walsall.

World Health Organization Europe. Davies E, Higginson IJ (eds) (2004). *Better Palliative Care for Older People.* WHO, Copenhagen.

Appendix **Useful organisations**

Action for Advocacy, PO Box 31856, Lorrimore Square, London
SE17 3XR. Tel: 020 7820 7868, Fax: 020 7820 9947
Email: info@actionforadvocacy.org.uk
Website: www.actionforadvocacy.org.uk

Action on Elder Abuse, Astral House, 1268 London Road, Norbury,
London SW16 4ER. Tel: 020 8765 7000, Fax: 020 8679 4074
Email: enquiries@elderabuse.org.uk
Website: http://www.elderabuse.org.uk

Age Concern England, Astral House, 1268 London Road,
London SW16 4ER.
Website: www.ageconcern.org.uk

British Geriatrics Society, Marjory Warren House, 31 St John's Square,
London EC1M 4DN. Tel: 020 7608 1369, Fax: 020 7608 1041
Email: general.information@bgs.org.uk
Website: www.bgs.org.uk

British Medical Association, BMA House, Tavistock Square, London
WC1H 9JP. Tel: 020 7387 4499, Fax: 020 7383 6400
Email: info.public@bma.org.uk
Website: www.bma.org.uk

Court of Protection, Archway Tower, 2 Junction Road, London N19 5SZ.
Tel: 020 7664 7300, Fax: 020 7664 7168
Email: custserv@guardianship.gsi.gov.uk
Website: www.guardianship.gov.uk

Dementia Services Development Centre, Stirling University, Iris
Murdoch Building, University of Stirling, Stirling, FK9 4LA, Scotland.
Tel: 01786 467740, Fax: 01786 466846
Website: www.dementia.stir.ac.uk

Department of Health (England), Richmond House, 79 Whitehall, London SW1A 2NS. Tel: +44 (0)20 7210 4850
Website: www.dh.gov.uk

Department of Health, Social Services and Public Safety (Northern Ireland), Castle Buildings, Stormont, BELFAST, BT4 3SJ.
Tel: 028 9052 0500
Email: webmaster@dhsspsni.gov.uk
Website: www.dhsspsni.gov.uk

General Medical Council, Regent's Place, 350 Euston Road, London NW1 3JN. Tel: 020 7189 5404, Fax: 020 7189 5401
Email: standards@gmc-uk.org
Website: www.gmc-uk.org

Health and Community Care, Scottish Government,
Tel: 08457 741 741 or 0131 556 8400
Email: ceu@scotland.gsi.gov.uk
Website: http://www.scotland.gov.uk

Health and Social Care, Welsh Assembly Government, Welsh Assembly Government, Cathays Park, Cardiff, CF10 3NQ. Tel: 0845 010 3300 (English) or 0845 010 4400 (Welsh)
Email: health.enquiries@wales.gsi.gov.uk
Website: www.wales.gov.uk

Help the Aged, 207–221 Pentonville Road, London N1 9UZ.
Tel: 020 7278 1114, Fax: 020 7278 1116
Email: info@helptheaged.org.uk
Website: www.helptheaged.org.uk

Independent Mental Capacity Advocacy Service, Department of Health, Wellington House, 133 Waterloo Road, London SE1 8UG.

Information Commissioner's Office – England, Wycliffe House, Water Lane, Wilmslow, Cheshire, SK9 5AF. Tel: 01625 54 57 45, Fax: 01625 524510
Website: www.ico.gov.uk

Information Commissioner's Office – Northern Ireland, 51 Adelaide Street, Belfast, BT2 8FE, Northern Ireland, Tel: 028 9026 9380, Fax: 028 9026 9388
Email: ni@ico.gsi.gov.uk

Information Commissioner's Office – Scotland, 28 Thistle Street, Edinburgh, EH2 1EN. Tel: 0131 225 6341, Fax: 0131 225 6989
Email: scotland@ico.gsi.gov.uk

Information Commissioner's Office – Wales, Cambrian Buildings, Mount Stuart Square, Cardiff, CF10 5FL. Tel: 029 2044 8044, Fax: 029 2044 8045
Email: wales@ico.gsi.gov.uk

Mental Welfare Commission for Scotland, K Floor, Argyle House, 3 Lady Lawson Street, Edinburgh EH3 9SH. Tel: 0131 222 6111, Fax: 0131 222 6112
Email: enquiries@mwcscot.org.uk
Website: http://www.mwcscot.org.uk

Nursing & Midwifery Council, 23 Portland Place, London W1B 1PZ. Tel: 020 7637 7181, Fax: 020 7436 2924
Website: www.nmc-uk.org

Official Solicitor of the Supreme Court, 81 Chancery Lane, London WC2A 1DD. DX 0012 London/Chancery Lane. Tel: 020 7911 7127, Fax: 020 7911 7105
Email: enquiries@offsol.gsi.gov.uk
Website: www.officialsolicitor.gov.uk

Official Solicitor of the Supreme Court for Northern Ireland, Royal Courts of Justice, PO Box 410, Chichester Street, Belfast BT1 3JF. Tel: 028 9023 5111, Fax: 028 9031 3793
Email: officialsolicitorsoffice@courtsni.gov.uk
Website: www.courtsni.gov.uk

Office of the Public Guardian, Archway Tower, 2 Junction Road, London N19 5SZ. Tel: 0845 330 2900, Fax: 0870 739 5780
Email: custserv@guardianship.gsi.gov.uk
Website: www.guardianship.gov.uk

Office of the Public Guardian, Scotland, Hadrian House, Callendar Business Park, Callendar Road, Falkirk, FK1 1XR. DX 550360 FALKIRK 3. Tel: 01324 678300, Fax: 01324 678 301
Email: opg@scotcourts.org.uk
Website: www.publicguardian-scotland.gov.uk

Patients Association, PO Box 935, Harrow, Middlesex HA1 3YJ.
Tel: 020 8423 9111, Fax: 020 8423 9119
Email: mailbox@patients-association.com
Website: www.patients-association.org.uk

Resuscitation Council (UK), 5th Floor, Tavistock House North, Tavistock
Square, London WC1H 9HR. Tel: 020 7388 4678, Fax: 020 7383 0773
Email: enquiries@resus.org.uk
Website: www.resus.org.uk

Royal College of General Practitioners, 14 Princes Gate, Hyde Park,
London SW7 1PU. Tel: 020 7581 3232, Fax: 020 7225 3047
Email: info@rcgp.org.uk
Website: www.rcgp.org.uk

Royal College of Nursing, 20 Cavendish Square, London W1M 0AB.
Tel: 020 7409 3333, Fax: 020 7647 3435
Website: www.rcn.org.uk

Royal College of Physicians, 11 St Andrew's Place, London NW1 4LE.
Tel: 020 7935 1174, Fax: 020 7487 5218
Website: www.rcplondon.ac.uk

Royal College of Physicians and Surgeons of Glasgow, 232–242 St Vincent
Street, Glasgow G2 5RJ. Tel: 0141 221 6072, Fax: 0141 221 1804
Website: www.rcpsglasg.ac.uk

Royal College of Physicians of Edinburgh, 9 Queen Street, Edinburgh
EH2 1JQ. Tel: 0131 225 7324, Fax: 0131 220 3939
Website: www.rcpe.ac.uk

Royal College of Surgeons of Edinburgh, Nicolson Street, Edinburgh
EH8 9DW. Tel: 0131 527 1600, Fax: 0131 557 6406
Email: information@rcsed.ac.uk
Website: www.rcsed.ac.uk

Royal College of Surgeons of England, 35–43 Lincoln's Inn Fields, London
WC2A 3PE. Tel: 020 7405 3474, Fax: 020 7831 9438
Website: www.rcseng.ac.uk

Index